Wyggeston and Queen Elizabeth I College

Please return the book on or before the last date shown below

USERS AND ABUSERS OF PSYCHIATRY

A Critical Look at Traditional Psychiatric Practice

LUCY JOHNSTONE

ROUTLEDGE

London and New York

First published 1989
by Routledge
11 New Fetter Lane, London EC4P 4EE

Simultaneously published in the USA and Canada
by Routledge
29 West 35th Street, New York, NY 10001

Reprinted 1995

Typeset in Times by Pat and Anne Murphy,
Highcliffe-on-Sea, Dorset
Printed and bound in Great Britain by
TJ Press (Padstow) Ltd, Padstow, Cornwall

British Library Cataloguing in Publication Data
A catalogue record for this book is available from the British Library

Library of Congress Cataloguing in Publication Data
A catalogue record for this book is available from the
Library of Congress

ISBN 0-415-02839-6 (hbk)
ISBN 0-415-02840-X (pbk)

Contents

To Roy and Mary McKay
my very dear grandparents
with love and admiration

Acknowledgements

My thanks to Helen Cottee, Tom Donald, Celia Kitzinger, Ron Lacey from MIND, Viv Lindow, Alan Moore from Men Overcoming Violence, Joan Neil, Dr Lawrence Ratna, Dr Dennis Scott, Lilly Stuart, Andy Treacher, David Winter; to my faithful panel of lay readers: Graham and Ann Johnstone, Canon Roy and Mrs Mary McKay, Stephen and Jessica Pidgeon, James Johnstone and Carole Cerasi; and to all the people whose stories appear in this book.

Glossary

A *psychiatrist* has a medical training and is able to prescribe drugs. Psychiatrists are at the head of the traditional psychiatric team.

A *clinical psychologist* is not medically trained, but has a degree in psychology followed by a post-graduate training course.

Psychotherapist is a general term for anyone of whatever profession who practises psychotherapy, the process of helping someone to understand and overcome their problems by encouraging them to talk through them in regular sessions, either on a one-to-one basis, or as a couple or a family, or in a group. The term 'counselling' describes the same process, perhaps carried out in a more low-key way. (More detailed descriptions of the different professions can be found in Chapter 7.)

I have used the term 'patient' throughout the book to refer to those people who are on the receiving end of psychiatric treatment. Although it is not a word I particularly like, I believe it conveys a more accurate impression of the position that these people find themselves in than euphemisms such as 'client' or 'resident'.

Names and identifying details of the people whose stories appear in this book have been changed.

Part One

THE PATIENTS

1

The story of a depressed housewife

This is the story of Elaine Jones, who is typical of very many women who break down and are taken into psychiatric hospitals.

Elaine's story

Elaine is 46, married with four children. Her husband is a van driver for a local firm, where she worked as a cleaner before her marriage.

Elaine is warm, outgoing, and intelligent, and cares very deeply for her family. Generally she seems to cope well with her life, which since her marriage has consisted mainly of looking after her husband and children. However, six months after the birth of her last child fifteen years ago, she suffered the first of recurring episodes of depression, which have often been so severe that she has tried to kill herself. She has had over twenty admissions to psychiatric hospitals, varying in length from a few days to several months. Her treatment has consisted mainly of medication; she has been prescribed twenty different drugs, and has been taking at least one of them ever since her first breakdown. She has also had ECT (electro-convulsive therapy). While in the occupational therapy department, she has followed programmes of cooking and sewing, pottery, and art. None of this has prevented her from breaking down again, sometimes only weeks or months after being discharged.

On Elaine's twenty-second admission, a new member of the psychiatric team, hearing that she had had a very unhappy childhood, suggested that she might benefit from a different treatment approach. This new team member was prepared to offer Elaine psychotherapy sessions to try and understand the background to and reasons for her depression. The consultant, who had had a lot of contact with Elaine over the past ten years, was not very keen on this idea. He was inclined to believe that Elaine was not so much depressed as seeking an escape from chores at home, and pointed out that a few weeks after admission she usually appeared looking perfectly cheerful, and asking to be discharged. However, he eventually agreed to the new plan.

Elaine, too, had mixed feelings about starting psychotherapy. She knew very little about it, and in any case she and her family had been told by her doctors that her depression was due to a recurrent illness. She found the idea of looking too closely at her feelings rather frightening. Nevertheless, she wanted to try anything that might help.

In the first session, Elaine started to reveal the depression behind the brave face that she felt compelled to put on for the world. Ever since childhood she had been known as the 'strong one', and she felt tremendously guilty about not being able to be strong for her family all the time. Although the battle was often horrific, she had forced herself to carry on through many bouts of depression without coming into hospital. Sometimes she had vomited with the strain of preparing herself for family gatherings, but not wanting to let people down, she somehow got through them without her social facade cracking. At other times, though, she reached the point where even washing a plate seemed like climbing a mountain, and she collapsed and retreated to bed in an extremity of exhaustion, guilt, and despair.

Elaine also described how hurt she was that others did not understand how she felt. Her brother slammed the telephone down on her one night when for once she rang for help. Tears came to her eyes as she recalled the incident. But she expressed nothing but gratitude to the hospital for taking her in so often. The consultant had insisted on discharging her once after a three-month stay when she had not improved at all, and although she had thought she would not be able to stand it, she had in fact struggled through in the end. At the time she had thought him harsh, but looking back she was grateful to him for his firmness.

In that initial session, Elaine also revealed for the first time the incident that had precipitated her first breakdown. She had been feeling very low after the birth of her third child, when some homeless relatives and their children arrived on the doorstep. She and her husband had felt obliged to take them in, and most of the burden of looking after two families in a medium-sized council house had fallen on Elaine's shoulders. The visiting husband started drinking heavily, and the whole family departed after six months without a word of thanks. Elaine broke down shortly afterwards.

In twice-weekly meetings over the next four months, Elaine and her therapist continued to trace the roots of her depression. A theme that emerged very strongly was the resentment and anger behind Elaine's guilt and depression. She had helped to set up a situation in which it was somehow always she who did the giving, while getting no acknowledgement from anyone else. For example, in the build-up to the present admission, her stepmother had invited an extra six relatives for Christmas lunch at Elaine's house. Since it had always been Elaine's task to cook the meal, she had felt unable to refuse or to ask for extra help. Her Christmas had been a nightmare of shopping, cooking, and organizing. Elaine's life was filled with similar incidents. Her sons expected dinner to be ready as soon as they came in, although sometimes they arrived hours late with no apologies. Her father and stepmother were offended if she did not visit them, and yet often neglected to visit her when she was in hospital. Even on her weekend leaves from hospital she rushed around doing household chores while the rest of the family had a lie-in. She described tearfully how it was always she who went forward to kiss her children and parents at visiting time, ask them how they were, and give them the cakes she had baked in occupational therapy during the day. 'Why can't it be the other way round for once?' she cried.

The irony was that Elaine's 'brave face' was too effective. Patients mistook her for a nurse and implied that she didn't really need to be in hospital, while her sister openly said that she was just looking for an escape from her responsibilities. Elaine feared that the hospital staff thought the same, though they denied it to her face. Elaine had set a trap for herself; she felt she had no right to protest or be dissatisfied, so she struggled on, putting on a façade which others were deceived

by, and then felt angry and hurt at being so badly misunderstood, as well as guilty at not being able to cope. She tried
to suppress these feelings too, and so the vicious circle
continued.

Elaine and her therapist started looking into her childhood
for the origins of this pattern. The accumulation of hurts,
resentments, and losses went back many years. Elaine was 9
when her mother died. Shortly afterwards Elaine's father
remarried, and two further children were born. Elaine and the
two boys from the first marriage were shunned, and although
still a child herself, Elaine had to bring up her younger
brothers. She was kept back from school to do the housework
and despatched to relatives to help out, while her half-sisters
had every attention and comfort. Elaine, known as the 'strong
one', was expected to cope with all this without acknowledgement, support, or affection, and as a young child she had little
option but to comply. It was very painful for Elaine to recall
these events from her past. At one point she cried out in
anguish, 'Why did they do it to me? I needed love too! Why
did they have everything and I had nothing?' and she wept
bitterly. But as the hurts were gradually released, she experienced the sensation of a hard lump in her chest slowly
dissolving.

Elaine and her therapist discussed the ways in which she was
still continuing her childhood role of serving others, bottling
up her feelings, having to be 'strong' and not having anything
for herself. On the one hand, she seemed to spend her life
apologizing and fighting for the right to exist. On the other, a
part of her was starting to say more strongly, as she put it,
'I'm *me*, I'm an individual — I'm not just a cook and wife
and mother! I've got to have some life of my own!'

Slowly, Elaine started to make changes in her life. She
resolved that this time she would not discharge herself from
hospital long before she was really recovered, telling the
doctors untruthfully that she was fine because she felt so guilty
at taking up their time and neglecting her home. She allowed
herself to let down her façade a little, and ask the staff for help
and support when she was at her worst. She was firmer with
people who questioned her need to be in hospital, whether they
were staff, patients, or family. Her therapist arranged a
different occupational therapy programme so that cooking
was replaced by more enjoyable and relaxing activities.

The major changes had to take place within her family. There were some successes. On weekend leave, instead of cleaning out the kitchen cupboards, she started to go on outings with her husband. She summoned up the courage to tell her brother how much his actions had hurt her, and although he was not very receptive, she found an unexpected ally in her sister-in-law. In fact, they discovered that they were both fed up with various aspects of Elaine's parents' behaviour, and decided to visit them less often even if there were complaints and 'bad atmospheres'.

However, Elaine was still very fragile, and often despaired of the possibility of changing entrenched patterns of behaviour in her own home. Her two daughters, who uncomplainingly took on the role of cleaning and caring for the men of the family during Elaine's admissions, had never given much trouble, but they, like Elaine, found it hard to break the habit of running round after everyone else. Her two sons resisted change very fiercely. Elaine asked for her husband's support in challenging the long-standing tradition that they contributed none of their earnings for food, keep, or laundry, and a furious row broke out. For once Elaine held her ground, only to be told by her sons that she was 'hysterical', 'crazy', and needed 'another spell in the loony bin'. Most hurtful of all, her husband changed sides and accused her of stirring up trouble and being too hard on young lads who deserved a bit of fun. Still fragile and unsure of her new self, Elaine was driven close to despair by such incidents. She felt it was desperately unfair that while everyone else was allowed to get angry and have their say, when she spoke up for once, instead of trying to soothe everyone else, she was labelled as 'crazy' and the whole family ranged themselves against her. Yet she now realized very clearly that her only hope of staying out of hospital was to bring about changes at home. Both options seemed so bleak that she sometimes contemplated running away and leaving the family, but they were her whole life and she felt she could never do it.

Elaine tried to explain some of this to her husband. He had coped valiantly with the children during her many admissions, refusing to have them put into care, and she deeply appreciated how much he had had to bear over the years. At the same time the changes in her were beginning to highlight severe difficulties in their relationship. She knew him well enough to sense that he was feeling very low himself, and his ulcers had flared up again. Yet he refused to confide in her, his GP, or anyone else. Nor would he come up to the hospital for a joint session, saying, 'The next thing, they'll put *me* in there too!'. When they made time to sit down quietly and talk, he would try hard to understand what she was going through, but in family crises he was as likely to shout at her as support her. He frequently exploded in violent rages. Elaine told her therapist, 'Sometimes I think *he* should be here talking to you, instead of me'.

Over the following weeks, Elaine needed a great deal of support, which she gained both from her therapist and from a small therapy group of other patients. Slowly, she increased in strength and confidence. Indeed, she said, 'If I'd had this sort of help fifteen years ago, I might not have needed to be on pills all this time'. But she couldn't afford to look back with regrets, because she knew the struggle to bring about changes in herself, her life and her family would continue for many months and need all her courage and determination. After a longer stay than most, she reached the point of being genuinely ready for discharge. She intended this admission to be her last one. Time will tell whether she succeeds.

Elaine's story is a clear illustration of many of the themes with which this book will be concerned. It can be understood and examined on various levels.

THE PSYCHOLOGICAL ANGLE

Let us look at Elaine's episodes of depression from a psychological point of view. Her psychotherapy gives us a way of understanding her depression as part of her whole person, of all of her past and present experiences and relationships, rather than just as an unpleasant recurring illness.

Clearly, Elaine was severely emotionally (and to some extent materially) deprived from a very young age. Not only did she miss out on the love, care, and attention that all children need, she was also expected to provide it for others — her younger brothers and other relatives. She was bearing adult responsibilities without getting the emotional nourishment that she needed for herself. Her parents seem to have justified this treatment by designating her as the 'strong one' who could cope with anything. Elaine learned to accept this view, which effectively stopped her from complaining or questioning the set-up. She too believed that she should be able to cope. In any case, she had very little choice in the matter.

Since the capacity to meet other people's needs depends on having had your own needs met in the first place, someone in Elaine's position is in constant danger of becoming emotionally overdrawn, as it were, and of not having the resources to cope with others' demands. Moreover, someone like Elaine is particularly likely to get into the situation where others are making a lot of demands, since the role of looking after others is one they have been trained in from childhood. As Elaine herself came to realize through her therapy, she had contributed to setting up a repetition of her childhood circumstances, and still felt she had no right to protest about it.

Obviously, a lifestyle based on such fragile foundations cannot continue indefinitely. There comes a point where so much more is being given out than is taken in that the whole system breaks down. Sometimes the event that is the 'last straw' seems fairly trivial. Since the family, psychiatric staff, and indeed the woman herself have usually subscribed to the myth of her as strong and capable, the sort of person who helps *others* with their problems, they are often at a loss to understand why a relatively minor incident precipitates such a severe reaction. They are unlikely to appreciate that from a psychological point of view, the breakdown can be understood as a cry for rest, care, and the replenishment of depleted resources, and as a desperate protest against an intolerable lifestyle.

The significance of the precipitating event for Elaine's first breakdown now becomes clearer. After the birth of her last child, she was fragile and vulnerable. At the same time, she was required to meet the needs of others — her baby and her existing family — and to push her own needs into the background. It was a repetition of her childhood predicament. For many women, made vulnerable by similar backgrounds, childbirth on its own is enough to trigger off what is usually described as 'post-natal depression', but often has its roots much further back. For Elaine, however, the problem was compounded by a whole extra set of demands from the relatives who came to stay. There was just too much weight on the wrong side of the fragile balancing act, and Elaine tipped over from 'strong one' to 'sick one'.

Real recovery from depression, as opposed to merely managing and containing it with medication, involved change on a whole-person level. Elaine had to find a way of completing the many unfinished events from her past that still haunted her. The major part of this work was done in the therapy sessions, where she was given permission to release the hurt and anger she had been carrying around for so many years. By shouting, weeping, and grieving, Elaine was able to work through and come to an acceptance of her past, and to liberate the energy that had been bound up in keeping all this pain bottled up inside. At the same time, she needed to fill her emptiness with support, under-standing, and care from her individual and group sessions. Her feelings had to be recognized and validated, not labelled and dismissed. Finally, she could turn to the task of redefining herself and her life.

Elaine's therapy also showed that her depression had to be understood, not just as part of a whole person, but as part of a whole system. She was involved in a network of relationships which included her husband, parents, children, brothers and sisters, friends, patients, and hospital staff, and many of the interactions between these people were actually helping to maintain her depression. For most of her fifteen-year career as a psychiatric patient, this system was stable, if uncomfortable. Various people continued to hurt and use her, Elaine continued to allow herself to be hurt and used, and the psychiatrists continued to admit her to hospital at regular intervals to continue the same treatment as before. Through her therapy, Elaine was made aware of this pattern and the way in which she had, in her own words, 'made a rod for my own back'. As she started to change her contribution to the pattern — for example, refusing to do her sons' laundry — other members of the system found that their roles were being challenged too. If, in certain instances, she was not willing to be the servant, they were no longer so clearly the masters. Change was forced upon them too.

When someone like Elaine starts off this process of change, two things characteristically occur. First, it becomes much less clear who really is the 'patient'. Elaine and her family had long ago accepted the doctors' definition of her as the 'sick one' in the family. However, as she began to make sense of her depression and climb out of the passive, suffering 'sick role' to become more active and assertive, the problems in the rest of the family came into clearer focus. Her husband, in particular, seemed to be or to become quite depressed in his own right. It began to look as if it had been part of Elaine's function to 'carry' the depression for both partners in the marriage. While she was the 'sick one', he could continue the familiar but limited role of strong, silent head of the family. As she changed and demanded more understanding and emotional support from him, it became apparent that he was completely unable to deal with his own or other people's feelings other than by blocking them off. Other members of the family had their difficulties too — the daughters tending to follow their mother's lead, and the sons to follow their father. In fact, it could be said that in some ways Elaine's depression had served the function of camouflaging the problems of the whole family.

The second characteristic occurrence is that there is strong resistance to change from other members of the system, who find themselves being challenged in very uncomfortable ways. Elaine's sons didn't want to do their own laundry; her husband was scared of acknowledging his own feelings; her brother was reluctant to admit that he had been hurtful. Although they would doubtless all have said they would do anything to cure the 'illness' which had brought the whole family such unhappiness, a view of her difficulties which included a critical look at their own contributions was not so welcome. In fact, their reaction was to try and push Elaine back into the 'sick role' by labelling her new and healthily assertive behaviour as 'hysterical' and 'crazy'. Thus their own investment in keeping her sick was revealed.

For Elaine, too, it was tempting to fall back into this familiar role, keep quiet, and struggle on as before, paying the price of needing future hospital admissions. Some psychiatric patients actually prefer to stay in the sick role, with the compensating benefit of avoiding painful conflict. Many others stay in the role that psychiatrists and other staff assign to them because they do not get the help they need to break out of it. Either way, a false solution, a kind of unhappy compromise, is reached. No one is especially happy, but on the other hand, everyone can avoid facing certain painful issues. In such cases, the unresolved problem tends to be passed on to reappear in future generations. This can be seen in Elaine's case. Elaine's daughters had learned to take over her role, stepping in to do the cooking, shopping, and cleaning for the whole family, including their grown-up brothers. Possibly they too had unfulfilled emotional needs because of their mother's depression and absences during their upbringing. Their compliant behaviour allowed the men of the family to act selfishly and ignore other people's rights and feelings. All the children were thus set up to repeat the pattern in their own families: the men prepared to exploit, and the women to allow themselves to be exploited. In this way, the sins of the fathers (and mothers) are visited upon the sons (and daughters).

THE MEDICAL ANGLE

Let us now look at the part played by the hospital and its staff in Elaine's story.

In fifteen years and twenty-two admissions to two different hospitals, Elaine came into contact with more than twenty psychiatrists, including three consultants, and a large number of nurses, occupational therapists, and other staff. Some of the psychiatrists saw her simply as the unfortunate victim of a recurrent illness which caused her to become depressed. Most of the others would have agreed, if asked, that childhood experiences and family relationships play a part in depression, but with little or no training in psychotherapy, they did not have the skills to work out how this might apply to Elaine. In this they were no wiser than Elaine herself, who hadn't realized how her upbringing was still affecting her and blamed herself for everything, and initially presented a picture of a happy family where only she was at fault. With a long list of other patients to be seen, it was easier for the psychiatrists to fall back on something they did know about: medical-style treatment consisting of diagnosis, hospitalization, and medication, all of which carried the implication that Elaine was suffering from some kind of mental illness. In Elaine's notes, the words 'depressive neurosis' or 'endogenous depression' appeared in the space left for diagnosis. Although details of Elaine's childhood were dutifully recorded by each of the many doctors who admitted her, no one was able to relate them to her current depression in a way that helped to make sense of it. Nor were the interactions between Elaine and her extended family investigated or discussed. In other words, Elaine's depression was treated, whether deliberately or in default of any alternative, not as part of a *whole person* and a *whole system*, but as an isolated phenomenon. Elaine and her family accepted the professional view that frequent admissions and permanent medication were the best hope of keeping it under control.

In fifteen years of pill-taking, Elaine had been prescribed the following drugs:

Stelazine	Tofranil
Largactil	Nardil
Melleril	Nomifensine
Procyclidine	Tranxene
Amitriptyline	Valium
Prothiaden	Mogadon
Tryptizol	Priadel
Tryptophan	Dothiepin

She had also had ECT (electro-convulsive therapy or electric shock treatment) whereby an electric current is passed through the brain simulating an epileptic fit.

Elaine also received treatment on what might be called a behavioural level, i.e. focusing quite simply on the activities, or behaviours, that she was unable to carry out. Here the equation seemed to be:

Problem: she says she can't cope with the cooking and shopping. *Solution:* make her do the cooking and shopping. Hence she was assigned to cooking programmes in occupational therapy, as well as art, pottery, and discussion groups.

Clearly, though, Elaine's physical treatment was not particularly successful. Her doctors might have argued that she would have been even worse off without medication, which at least cured her for a time, although Elaine herself said that she was nearly always aware of depression lurking in the background. But there seems to have been general resignation to the fact that she would need to come into hospital regularly, and to be supported with medication — supervised in fortnightly or monthly outpatient appointments — in between. Patients do not have the right to read their medical notes, and no one may quote from them without the permission of the health authority. However, perhaps some fictional examples based on typical real-life extracts will serve to illustrate how the 'medical model' approach works in practice.

In cases such as Elaine's, the accumulation of notes and letters tends to follow a predictable sequence. There will be a pile of memos from psychiatrist to general practitioner monitoring progress and making minor adjustments to medication following the fifteen-minute appointments, along the lines of:

Dear Michael, re: Mrs Elaine Jones, I saw this patient of yours today in my outpatient clinic. Her depression is improved and she is doing fairly well on Dothiepin 150 mgs nocte. I have suggested she reduces the Tranxene to 15 mgs daily. I will see her again in two weeks' time.

After some months or years of ringing the changes in this way, with no substantial change in the patient's condition, a slight note of desperation may creep in, although the remedy is still to prescribe more of the same treatment rather than revise the treatment approach itself. One might then see:

Dear Michael, I saw Mrs Elaine Jones who is still complaining of severe depression, with associated early morning wakening, lethargy, and loss of appetite. Although I appreciate she has not done very well on tricyclics, I thought it might be worth starting her on Tofranil, possibly combined with ECT and/or admission at a later date if her condition seems to warrant it.

Or there may be a bald statement about recent stresses, without any suggestion that it might be useful or relevant to discuss the meaning and implications of these with the patient: 'Her son has recently left home to start a college course, and her elderly mother is ill. I will be seeing her again on . . . .' At this stage, there may be some grasping of straws, at the possibility that another physical cause will be found so that she can be put right, perhaps: 'She seems to be worse pre-menstrually, and I wonder if it would be worth referring her to Dr Smith for possible hormonal therapy.' Even a psychological hypothesis may be put forward, usually to be dismissed: 'One suspects that her marriage plays some part in her depression, but I am doubtful about the likelihood of change in that area.' A male psychiatrist's identification with the husband who also has to deal with this awkward woman may be revealed by such phrases as, 'Mr Jones has put up with his wife's outbursts with remarkably good humour over the years.'

Finally, a note of persecution creeps in. The patient has obstinately refused to get better, and someone who started off five years ago as 'this very pleasant lady' may end up as 'this difficult woman' or worse.

If we look at the effect of the medical model approach on Elaine's depression, we can see that one result of ignoring the whole-person, whole-system approach is to deny that her feelings and reactions have any validity. It is not that she has reason to be depressed, or exhausted, or tearful — these are merely symptoms of her illness. This effectively traps her in her situation. She does not strive for change, because important professionals who know about these matters have defined her problem in such a way that she is prevented from realizing that change is necessary. Her part is to comply obediently with the treatment that they prescribe. Indeed, the underlying message of giving pills to a patient is, 'Let *me* diagnose and treat this problem for you. Follow my instructions and you will be better'. This may be very appropriate for earache or 'flu — but for someone like Elaine, it is not only not helpful, it is actually harmful. The final irony is that she even thanks the hospital for their treatment, and feels especially grateful to the consultant who discharged her, protesting, despairing, and unhelped, back to the very situation that was contributing to her problems in the first place.

As we have seen, the illness model also reinforces the family's natural tendency to exempt themselves from playing any part in Elaine's depression. Their need to see the entire problem as located in Elaine and her 'illness' is legitimized.

To summarize, Elaine's treatment not only failed to address the wider issues at stake, but actually ensured that they would not be addressed. It not only failed to help Elaine, it actually perpetuated her difficulties. Indeed, one could go further and say that the medical model approach not only perpetuates, but actually creates, the difficulties it purports to solve — because as we have seen, Elaine's children are set up to carry the problem down the generations.

There are thousands of Elaines in Britain's psychiatric hospitals. Indeed, I have chosen her story because it is one of the most common. This is not to say that Elaine would have suffered the same fate everywhere. The standards of psychiatric practice vary, and there are some excellent wards, centres, and hospitals which offer a very good service to their patients. Nevertheless, the fact that the combined efforts of more than twenty psychiatrists and many other staff over fifteen years failed even to start to help Elaine make sense of her depression indicates that she was not just the victim of an unfortunate oversight. Nor is such treatment found only in the more backward asylums; most of Elaine's admissions were to a modern psychiatric unit in a district general hospital. She had in fact received fairly standard psychiatric care as practised in the majority of hospitals in this country. If this is so, how and why does it happen?

Part of the answer lies in the training that doctors, nurses, and other psychiatric staff receive. Contrary to popular belief, most of these professionals are *not* primarily trained to understand people and their problems. Doctors are mainly trained to diagnose and prescribe, nurses to manage wards, occupational therapists to run pottery and discussion groups, and so on. If they do have additional skills in counselling or psychotherapy, these will probably have been gained on courses taken voluntarily after training, or picked up on the job.

Another factor is that even the best efforts are compromised by working within the psychiatric system. Some of Elaine's nurses spent hours talking with her and some of her doctors would doubtless have learned to understand her much better had they not been obliged to move on every six months to fulfil their training requirements, or had they had more time and supervision. However, the overall policy towards a patient tends to sabotage whatever more constructive work may be carried out, unofficially, by staff lower down the hierarchy. By the time someone gets to be a 'known depressive', usually about their second or third admission, the chances of them getting different treatment from before become fairly remote — partly because success would challenge the correctness of the original decisions. As we saw, the consultant was reluctant for Elaine to have psychotherapy, even though his own efforts had not met with notable success. So, while individual members of staff may be trying their best to understand the patient as a person in a difficult situation, their efforts will be undermined by the overall message that she or he is 'ill'.

Finally, the 'illness' model enables the psychiatric staff themselves, like Elaine's family, to avoid facing and sharing the enormous amount of pain that Elaine and others like her are carrying around inside them. They can distance themselves from their own hurts, fears, and frustrations, which might otherwise be stirred up. They do not have to confront the difficult questions that Elaine's anguish might raise about their own attitudes, families, beliefs, roles, and the society in which these things take place.

THE 'SEX ROLE' ANGLE

Let us look at Elaine's depression from yet another perspective; that of sex role expectations.

Elaine, like 5 out of every 7 people admitted to psychiatric hospital ever year,[1] is a woman. One way of viewing her problems, and those of many of her fellow-patients, is that she was caught in the contradictions of the traditional female role.

Part of Elaine's dilemma was that she was expected to give without receiving enough in return, leading to a build-up of need and resentment. Believing that she ought to be able to cope with this, she blamed all her failures on herself, without questioning the role that had been thrust upon her. This was not just Elaine's particular misfortune, although she had an especially rigorous training in it. Women in general, especially those of Elaine's generation, are expected to spend their lives giving to others — their husbands, children, and extended families. They are defined not as individuals, but in relation to others — wife, mother. Even outside the family, the jobs that involve most in terms of giving, and return least in terms of salary and status, are held by women — nurses, domestics, secretaries. When Elaine cried out, 'I'm not just a wife and mother, I'm me! I'm an individual! I've got to have some life of my own!' she was speaking not just for herself, but for her whole sex. The women who break down and come into psychiatric hospitals tend to be those who have adopted the traditional woman's role most completely.

Behind every woman trapped in her sex role, there is a man trapped in his. The partner who presents to the psychiatric services is nearly always the woman, since women in trouble characteristically become unable to *act* but are overwhelmed by their *feelings*. Men, on the other hand, who are generally far less in touch with their *feelings*, but are freer to *act* in the world, are more likely to deal with distress by such means as drinking, violence, and delinquency, and ultimately to end up in prison rather than psychiatric hospitals. They may also manifest distress in physical illnesses. While Elaine followed the woman's pattern, her husband was prone to violent outbursts, and had severe ulcers. As Elaine progressed, his inability to deal with his feelings in any other way became very apparent. His male conditioning did not equip him to deal with years of strain or to meet his wife on an emotional level. He was trapped too.

Again, the hospital served to reinforce rather than challenge these complementary roles. As far as Elaine's husband was concerned, no attempt was made to allow for his feelings over fifteen difficult years, to encourage him to express them or to see his wife's desperation as anything more than the symptom of an illness. His part in the treatment was limited to meeting the doctors from time to time to discuss what was going to be done to his wife next.

As for Elaine, the hospital's message was quite clear. She was supposed to be able to cope with all her domestic duties without complaining. Even in hospital she was assigned to programmes of cooking and sewing, the clear implication being that this was her job. No one, including Elaine herself, questioned the assumption that this desperate woman should force herself to make flans and cakes while fighting off suicidal despair, and should dutifully present them to her family each evening. Indeed, successful treatment was defined in terms of her being able to return home and uncomplainingly continue the same activities. Obediently following this regime on the advice of experts, Elaine felt she had no one but herself to blame when she still did not get better, and yet more guilt was added to her despair. In this too she was following the pattern of the rest of her sex, who characteristically blame themselves, their inadequacy, their weakness, their stupidity, or their fat thighs, rather than question the obligation to meet these standards in the first place.

As in Elaine's family, hospital staff too often resist healthy assertiveness in a truly recovering patient. Someone who sits miserably but quietly in a corner, taking their medication regularly, is easier to deal with than someone who is prepared to disagree, protest, and complain. Staff may show their resistance in the same way as Elaine's family did — by pushing her back into the 'sick role'. Patients are likely to acquire labels like 'aggressive' and 'paranoid' if their behaviour becomes too challenging.

What might be called the 'depressed housewife' syndrome, with variations, makes up the everyday bread-and-butter work of psychiatry. The unlucky ones will be getting exactly the same kind of treatment.

If traditional psychiatry fails these women so badly, as I believe it does, then it does little better with other categories of patient — people who have acquired the labels of schizophrenia, obsessional-compulsive disorder, manic-depression, anorexia, and so on. Yet 79,000 beds, or about one-third of all NHS beds, are filled with psychiatric patients,[2] at a cost of several hundred pounds a week, and to keep them there without actually helping them is profoundly depressing and demoralizing for the staff. I have indicated some of the reasons why this state of affairs continues. A fuller answer takes us on to the rest of the book.

2

The Rescue Game

There are many misconceptions about psychiatric patients. Surveys consistently show that the general public believe they are unpredictable, potentially dangerous, and likely to commit violent and sexual crimes, particularly against children.[1] They are feared, distrusted, and disliked even more than the mentally handicapped, ex-prisoners, and alcoholics, who are the other least popular groups in society.[2] This damaging and inaccurate picture is heavily reinforced by the media, where headlines like 'Ex-mental patient sought by police' and 'Mad axeman kills two' are never balanced by more positive reports ('Ex-mental patient elected mayor' or 'Former patient rescues drowning girl'). In fact, only a very small minority of psychiatric patients is violent or dangerous in any way at all. You are more likely to get beaten up in your local pub than on a psychiatric ward. Again, the majority are there not because they are 'ill' or 'mad', but for a variety of other reasons — relationship difficulties, social problems, lack of anywhere else to go. All these may add up to loneliness, anxiety, or unhappiness, but not necessarily to what most people would view as an illness.

Patients are usually categorized according to medical diagnosis. The main division is psychotics (people who are out of touch with reality, or in a layperson's terms 'mad') versus neurotics. Under the first heading come diagnoses like schizophrenia, manic depression, and paranoia. Under the second heading would come agoraphobia, obsessional disorder, most cases of depression and anxiety, and many others. In order to get a clearer picture of what actually goes on in psychiatric hospitals, I propose to look at groups of patients not according to their diagnosis, but according to how they use the hospital and how the hospital characteristically responds.

1. There is a group of people who are asking for help with problems that are really marital or family issues. Elaine Jones is an obvious example.

2. There are people who ask for help with problems which, while still involving those around them, are not primarily to do with current marital or family relationships. An example might be someone who is bereaved, or who is a victim of rape or incest, or has had an accumulation of stressful life events.

3. There are other people who, usually for lack of alternative options or more appropriate forms of help, choose the career of psychiatric patient in order to escape painful situations in their lives.

4. There are those who use the hospital mainly to meet social or economic needs, perhaps because they are lonely and isolated, or have nowhere to go, or want to get a doctor's recommendation for council housing.

5. Hospitals may also be used for what is often called 'time out'. For example, an exhausted mother might come in for a break, or an unruly adolescent might be admitted for a week mainly to relieve his parents.

6. There is a group of people who are suffering from conditions of definitely physical origin, such as senile dementia, Huntington's Chorea, and severe head injury.

7. Finally, there are more extreme examples of the first category, where family relationships are so intense and entangled that one person in the system breaks down very severely.

Obviously these divisions are very rough, and many people will cut across several of them. There are typical diagnoses for some of the categories — schizophrenia is often the choice for the seventh group — but by using these categories rather than medical diagnoses as a guide, I hope to show what the psychiatric hospital actually does in response to people's overt or covert requests.

PEOPLE WHO ARE ASKING FOR HELP WITH PROBLEMS THAT ARE REALLY MARITAL OR FAMILY ISSUES

The 'depressed housewife' is the classic example of this type. She may be middle or working class, and may be treated as an in- or out-patient, producing many variations on the same theme. Let us look briefly at another depressed housewife fifteen years on.

Susan's story

Susan Smith is 58, a frail, timid, anxious-looking woman. She has been in and out of hospital with a diagnosis of depression for many years. Her admissions have usually been precipitated by complaints from her husband, Bill, that she is not keeping up with the household chores. He makes an outpatient appointment for her and brings her along, complaining forcefully about this and various other 'symptoms' such as her irrational fear that he is about to have an affair. She looks nervous and tearful, agrees she is depressed, and is admitted and medicated.

After many years of this treatment, a discussion in the ward round (the weekly meeting where staff meet to review patients' progress) led to a different attempt to help. The psychiatrist had been trying to avoid having to admit Susan by sending a community nurse to visit her home and instruct her in cooking and cleaning. This had not worked. At the most recent outpatient appointment, Bill angrily insisted that his wife needed to be kept in hospital for the rest of her life. However, the nurses commented that as soon as she arrived on the ward, Susan brightened up, settled in extremely happily, and showed no signs of depression. The clear indication was that the problem lay in the marital situation rather than simply in an illness suffered by Susan. A member of the team agreed to see the couple, not, this time, to pass a medical judgement on the wife, but to find out more about the marital relationship.

There were two sessions, both dominated by Bill. This large, well-built man loudly accused his thin, timorous wife of underfeeding him, of neglecting the housework, and of having irrational fears about his being unfaithful. He addressed the therapist condescendingly as 'dear' and demanded to know what she was going to do to improve the situation. The therapist, feeling rather overpowered, tried to point out that change would have to come from them as a couple, and that Susan might have her point of view too. But Susan, who sat in tremulous silence throughout these outbursts, could not take advantage of this invitation to voice her opinions. She seemed to have been completely cowed by years of submission and the therapist found out that she was fighting Susan's battle for her rather than helping her to fight it for herself. Meanwhile Bill frustrated all attempts to get him to listen to his wife by interrupting and loudly insisting that he had always tried every possible way to help. The therapist was only able to claim the limited success of blocking his demand that Susan should be locked away for good.

Here again we can see how medicalizing a relationship problem heavily reinforced the unhealthy aspects of the marriage — the husband's bullying dominance, which was the counterpart to his wife's cowering submission. If the problem had been seen in a whole-person, whole-system way right back when it started, it might have been possible to do some constructive work with the couple. Alternatively, if the hospital had refused to get involved at all, the resulting crisis might have forced change to occur. But by taking an unhappy middle line, defusing each periodic crisis by admitting Susan without actually taking any steps to deal with the underlying causes, the hospital played a crucial role in helping to maintain this destructive relationship exactly as it was. It was the necessary third player in this unhappy game.

Again, the values of the traditional woman's role were accepted without question and reinforced by the treatment, albeit in a slightly more progressive guise in later years (home visits by a nurse rather than automatic admission). The husband's complaints were accepted at face value, although it emerged in the sessions that one reason for Susan's so-called irrational fear of his being unfaithful was his continual threat to be exactly that if she did not pull herself together. Indeed, the therapist strongly suspected that he was already having affairs, and that his demands for his wife's hospitalization coincided with times when it would be convenient to have her out of the way. However, by this time the situation was too entrenched for change. Susan had lost all powers of opposition, and indeed usually entered the more congenial world of hospital very happily. She narrowly missed becoming one of the long-stay patients whose world is bounded by the grounds of a large Victorian asylum, where years of case notes slowly accumulate in the files. But perhaps, after so many years of admissions, this might have been the happiest solution for her.

THE RESCUE GAME

There are two predominant models or ways of viewing mental distress in psychiatry, one official and one unofficial. The first is the medical model, and the second might be called the 'pull-yourself-together' approach. They combine very destructively to take away responsibility from the patient, and then blame the patient for his or her helplessness. We saw with Elaine and Susan how the medical view initially encouraged them and their relatives to see them as helpless victims of an illness unconnected to the rest of their lives, which meant that the hospital had to step in and take responsibility for them. Logically, when this fails to help, as it inevitably does, the conclusion should be either that the illness is more severe or complex than had at first appeared, or that something else is going on. In general hospitals, patients do not get blamed for suffering from incurable illnesses or being misdiagnosed. In psychiatric hospitals, however, the suspicion that a psychological element is involved tends to manifest itself in a gradual switch from pitying to blaming the patient. She or he turns from 'mad' to 'bad' and comes to acquire one of the many diagnostic labels reserved for people whom the staff do not know how to help: hysterical, attention-seeking, manipulative, immature, inadequate, aggressive, histrionic. At this point, the patient may be abruptly discharged. They are then in a much worse state than before admission. They have been encouraged to hand over control and responsibility to the hospital and to depend on it for a solution, and have then been blamed for the hospital's failure to provide one. What they *are* left with is the original problem plus confusion, a sense of failure, possible dependence on medication, and a psychiatric label.

The process can be illustrated by a concept from the school of therapy called Transactional Analysis. Transactional Analysis analyses many of the interactions between people as games, with predictable outcomes, in which set roles are adopted by the participants. One common example is the Rescue Game, in which the two players take turns to adopt the three main roles of Rescuer, Persecutor, and Victim.

'Rescuing' occurs when one person needs help and another person tries to help them. The Rescuer, however, fundamentally believes that people cannot really be helped, and cannot help themselves either. The corresponding position of the Victim (or patient) is, 'I'm helpless and hopeless — try and help me'. The Rescuer responds to this challenge by stepping in and taking over responsibility for the Victim. Rescuing does not work and the Rescuer soon begins to feel angry with the Victim for being so helpless and hopeless and switches to Persecuting or punishing ('This manipulative patient . . .'). Or the Rescuer may end up being Persecuted by the Victim, who gets angry at being treated as less than equal, and may get his or her own back by making awkward demands, taking up staff time, and so on. Or, like Elaine, the patient may Rescue the staff by pretending to be better. (Rescuing was, of course, a lifelong pattern for Elaine.) The theory says that each player will occupy every position in the game at some time.

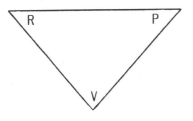

Figure 1   The drama triangle[3]

What the three positions have in common is that none of them can be a basis for relating to others as equals. You are either all-powerful or helpless. Some careers — nursing, medicine, the helping professions in general — are particularly suited to those who wish to play a lifelong game of Rescue. The medical profession, with its emphasis on power, status, and specialized knowledge, provides an excellent basis for Rescuing if that is what a person wants to do.

In psychiatry, the switch from Rescuer to Persecutor, from 'This patient is mad' to 'This patient is bad' is seen all the time. Some patients present themselves as Victims at first assessment. Some are pushed into the Victim role by the process of medicalizing their problems and gradually become more helpless and dependent on the psychiatric system, which in its turn gradually becomes more Persecutory as harsher remedies are tried out.

The same pattern can be seen on a global level. For example, it is increasingly recognized that simply flying in huge quantities of food to famine regions does not, in the long term, alleviate starvation. Local food prices fall, farmers go bankrupt, and the population gets dependent on external forms of aid. Real solutions depend on providing the kind of aid that enables people to develop their own skills and resources so that they can help themselves.

This is not to say that Rescuing is always inappropriate. In emergencies — after an overdose, say, or in the worst stages of famine — it may be necessary for someone else to take total responsibility for a short while. But in the long term any successful attempt to help people change needs to be based on a treatment contract drawn up by both parties as equal and responsible agents. This flies in the face of all the usual assumptions about the capabilities of those who are called mentally ill. There will be further discussion of this issue later — but in the meanwhile, the story of Sam Green illustrates some of these themes.

Sam's story

Sam Green was 60 and happily married with two grown stepchildren when he began to be terrified of getting cancer.

He had always been gentle, sensitive, and rather over-concerned about his health, but the phobia of cancer quickly grew out of all reasonable proportions. He was unable to go to work and paced around the house all day, checking himself for lumps which might be tumours. When his wife found him ringing the vet at midnight to complain that the cat had cancer, she and the GP agreed that it was time to call a psychiatrist.

The psychiatrist noted that there was a family history of cancer. Sam's mother had died of cancer of the throat — the part of his body that he was most worried about. Instead of following up this clue, she arranged for him to have ECT. This made him much more agitated. His sons complained that he was too much for his rather frail wife to cope with and Sam was therefore admitted to hospital and tried on a total of fifteen different drugs over the next six months.

Sam presented the staff with great problems. He constantly accosted nurses and doctors in the corridors to complain of aches and pains and to demand medical investigations which were always negative. Since no clear management plan had been drawn up — he had been admitted as a result of pressure from his sons, rather than as a response to any request from him — the nursing staff were unsure what they were supposed to be doing with him. They tried offering reassurance, which worked for a maximum of ten minutes. The occupational therapists tried to distract him with other activities, which was hard work and not usually very effective. A succession of junior doctors tried to resist his demands for more physical investigations and explained how anxiety was causing many of his symptoms, with equally little result. Meanwhile, in response to reports of the situation in the ward round, the consultant continued to ring the changes with tranquillizers and anti-depressants. On the whole this made him worse since many of the side effects, such as a dry mouth, were interpreted by Sam as sure signs of cancer.

Sam became increasingly frustrated and angry at being treated as mentally ill instead of having his supposed cancer investigated properly. His complaints became more persistent and soon there were no activities that he felt well enough to join in with. In other words, he started to Persecute the staff in response to the consultant's failed Rescue. The consultant, in her turn, completed his transformation from 'mad' to 'bad' by suggesting that he should be discharged. She was Persecuting him for not getting better by dismissing him unhelped and labelled as a bad patient. This was the situation after four months in hospital.

What no one had been able to do was to discover the meaning of Sam's fear in the context of him as a whole person living within a whole system of relationships. One of the staff was keen to explore Sam's fears along these lines and asked the consultant for permission to do this.

It was not at all easy to work with Sam. Always rather reserved and passive, his hospital treatment had confirmed an attitude of resentful helplessness in him. He was reluctant to communicate with the therapist except by relating a string of complaints about his supposed cancer. Given that Sam was desperate, resistant to suggestions, and unused to putting his feelings into words, the therapist decided to use some techniques from the Gestalt approach to therapy. This, in contrast to standard verbal psychotherapy, advocates 'doing' rather than 'talking about', and bringing issues into the here-and-now rather than having a discussion about what has happened in the past. Thus, having established that Sam had been

27

extremely close to his mother, and suspecting that he had not fully mourned her death, the therapist invited Sam to imagine his mother sitting in the chair opposite him and to tell her how very much he missed her. Hesitantly Sam did this. Then he told her how bitterly he regretted not being kinder to her before she died, adding, 'I sometimes wish I could die too so I could join you'. Tears came to his eyes and he sat in silence for a long while. Finally he was able to take the therapist's gentle suggestion that he should say goodbye to his mother for the last time.

It looked as if Sam's cancer phobia might be expressing his close identification with his mother and his desire still to be with her, even to the point of joining her in death. But Sam's fears and behaviour were unchanged after this piece of work. Several sessions later the therapist, unsure how else to help, invited Sam to try another Gestalt exercise and to have a conversation with the supposed cancer as if it was sitting in the room with him. Taking up his rather bizarre suggestion, Sam asked the cancer why it was attacking and trying to kill him. Directed to move into the opposite chair and speak for the cancer, he found himself answering forcefully that he didn't care about Sam, and he was going to overwhelm Sam and kill him and nothing was going to stop him. Sam threatened to cut the cancer out — but it replied that it would just come back in a different place. A conversation developed between Sam, scared but still struggling, and the hard conviction of the invading, destructive cancer.

According to Gestalt theory symptoms can be understood as rejected parts of oneself which reappear in a frightening and unrecognizable form. Speaking as the symptom, whether it is a phobia, a panic attack, a pain, or whatever, is the first step towards owning it as part of oneself and listening to the message it has to convey. Ultimately, so the theory goes, if the message is understood, the rejected aspect can be reintegrated, leading to greater wholeness.

What all this meant in Sam's case became clearer when the therapist, acting on the assumption that the cancer represented an important but rejected part of Sam, asked him to say to it, 'I admire you because . . .' and complete the sentence in his own way. Startled but compliant, Sam responded, 'I admire you because . . . you're strong and determined and you don't give up', and looked very surprised at what had come out of his mouth.

At this point, several pieces of the jigsaw began to fall into place. The qualities that were conspicuously lacking in Sam were strength, determination, and forcefulness. He sat back helplessly and allowed other people to make decisions for him, a pattern that had started in the relationship with his over-concerned mother and was reinforced by many aspects of his hospital treatment. He badly needed to integrate the more assertive side of himself, which at present only appeared in his behaviour as complaining and Persecuting, and in his symptoms, it seemed, as an invading cancer. But this threw Sam into a terrible dilemma. He had previously helped his therapist to describe and list the common characteristics of those family members who had succumbed to cancer. Sam saw them as soft, gentle, and kind-hearted — qualities that he valued highly and shared with his mother — although they were also rather weak. On the other hand, he saw the relatives who didn't get cancer as strong but hard, callous, and crafty. For Sam there seemed to be no mid-point which would allow him to be strong enough to avoid getting cancer without turning into the sort of person he feared and despised. This way of viewing the world in extremes very often underlies psychological problems. There are many people who fear that if they stop being martyrs they will instantly turn into domineering harridans; or that if they stop being sexless they will become nymphomaniacs; or that there is no mid-point between passivity and aggression.

Understanding Sam's problem better enabled a consistent treatment plan to be drawn up for him. While he continued to work with his therapist, the nurses showed him how to be more direct, outspoken, and assertive. They helped him decide how he could continue this behaviour on weekend leave in small but important ways — for example, asking his son to return a borrowed coat — and praised him for his successes.

Some small improvements were seen, but Sam was still very stuck. The whole-person view of his difficulties was much clearer now; but the whole system approach had been neglected. So, finally, what should have happened right at the beginning was arranged, and one of the nurses went to visit Sam's wife. This intelligent and thoughtful woman was able to give a very clear picture of the development of Sam's fears in the context of his relationships — far clearer than any put together by the professional staff. Thinking the whole matter over, she had realized how much she, fifteen years older than Sam, had taken over his mother's role when they married shortly after the latter's death. She had been very happy to carry on the pattern of looking after him and taking most of the decisions for both of them until her failing sight and increasing frailty had upset the routine. Far from stepping in to compensate, Sam had responded to the threatened loss of his second mother with panic and helplessness. If his wife fell and hurt her arm one day, he was quite likely to have a similar accident himself the next day, and retreat to bed demanding to be looked after. Sam's wife wanted him back and was quite willing to care for him as much as her physical condition permitted. Obviously, though, Sam needed help to come to terms with the independence that was being thrust on him so late in life, and this too became part of the nursing plan for him.

It would be misleading to imply that Sam's rehabilitation was easy. In fact, it was an uphill task for all the staff, and there was a predictable relapse when the time came to discharge him and break his dependence on the hospital. Six months later he was still complaining of various aches and pains. On the credit side, he had not needed readmission, his fear of cancer had receded, and he was taking a reasonable amount of responsibility at home.

Sam's story, like Elaine's, shows very clearly that neurotic symptoms are over-determined. In other words, there is rarely a single, straightforward cause. Instead there is a complicated web of meanings, all of which are contributing to the symptom and have to be unravelled. This needs to be done by looking at the whole person (in this case, Sam's personality and beliefs) as part of a whole system of relationships (i.e. Sam's way of relating to his mother, his wife, and the staff). If this is done successfully, then not only does the symptom fade, but the patient has a chance to achieve greater insight and wholeness by understanding and integrating the symptom's message. This happened to a certain extent with Sam. His fear of cancer receded, and he also learned to come to terms with his mother's death and to be a little more assertive.

In contrast, the orthodox medical approach aims to eliminate symptoms rather than understand their message. Sam viewed his cancer as an alien force to be cut out with knives if necessary.

In rather the same way, Sam's fear and Elaine's depression were seen by the doctors as things to be controlled and suppressed. But since Sam's fear and Elaine's depression had important messages to convey, they did not go away. In fact, the drugs' side-effects made Sam more anxious, while the underlying message of pill-prescribing — that the patient should rely on the doctors for a solution and comply with their instructions — fostered his passivity and dependence.

The commonest way to try to eliminate symptoms is by prescribing drugs. The drawback to this is, as patients often say, 'The pills make you *feel* better but they don't solve the problem'.

In more extreme cases, more extreme steps are taken. It is not known exactly how ECT (passing an electric current through the brain) works, but patients do sometimes report that they feel better afterwards, and ECT is seen as the treatment of choice in many cases of severe depression. And as a very last resort a leucotomy, the severing of nerve fibres in the brain, is occasionally carried out. The flaw in all these treatments is the assumption that removing the symptom is the same as solving the problem. Since this is not the case, repeated changes of drugs and rounds of ECT may be necessary even if the initial result is good, and this increases the likelihood of unpleasant side-effects and even permanent neurological damage. (These issues will be considered in detail in Chapter 9.) Moreover, because real healing has not taken place, patients may be unable to break their dependence on whatever is keeping them going — drugs, hospital admissions, or ECT — and become increasingly reliant on props that are steadily undermining their power to direct and control their own lives.

Physical treatments are not always either useless or harmful. Medication can be very valuable to tide someone over a crisis, or to provide a desperately needed breathing space, or as part of a properly thought-out treatment plan that takes all aspects of a patient's life into consideration. Far too often, though, medication and/or ECT are prescribed routinely and immediately as the main and often the only attempt at treatment. Moreover, this often happens without asking the patient whether she or he wants this kind of treatment and without giving any information about side-effects. Typically one of the doctors will say in the ward round, 'She seems a bit agitated, I thought we might try her on some X'. X will be written up on the drug chart, and the patient will be handed the appropriate dose by a nurse at the evening drug round. Protest or refusal is the quickest way of getting yourself labelled as a difficult patient — partly because it highlights the poverty of responses that psychiatric staff can make to psychological distress. If a patient will not take the pills, what else can be offered?

We have seen how the medical approach not only fails to promote the attitudes which would lead to a genuine solution to psychological problems, but actually undermines them. It has the same effect on alternative treatment approaches. By the time Elaine, Susan, and Sam reached their respective therapists, a great deal of energy needed to be expended on undoing the effects of their medical treatment so far (Sam's and Susan's increased passivity; Elaine's and her family's view of her depression as a recurring illness) before the original problem could be tackled at all. In Susan's case, it was too late. With Sam and Elaine, the danger was that the therapeutic work would be undermined by contradictory messages from the rest of the hospital, for example, that Elaine would continue to be instructed to work hard at her cooking programme although her therapist was encouraging her to have more time for herself; or that Sam would be Persecuted for trying out his new assertive behaviour on the ward. The split in the treatment approaches can come to mirror the split in the patient ('Should I be spending my whole life looking after others or not?'; 'Perhaps it is bad to stand up for myself'). If the external split — the split in the treatment approaches — is not resolved, then the split within the patient is unlikely to be resolved either. Thus, genuine attempts at a whole person, whole system approach are undermined by the context in which they take place. The patient ends up confused, while the therapist feels unsupported and alone.

In Sam's case there was good co-operation between the therapist and the nursing staff, although neither side was successful in requesting that his medication be stopped, and the outcome was reasonably good. What would have happened otherwise? The medical approach had encouraged this already dependent man to rely on the hospital for answers, and when these were not forthcoming had Persecuted him for his increased helplessness. His family too, were getting more and more irritated by his complaints, and he was in danger of being shuttled back and forwards between the two systems indefinitely, with a vicious circle building up as he became even more angry and helpless. One possible eventual outcome would have been rejection by both hospital and family, and entrance into a state of final helplessness as a long-stay patient on a back ward in a nearby asylum. Alternatively he might genuinely have developed a fatal cancer. There is an increasing amount of evidence that the mind plays an important part in determining who succumbs to cancer, and cancer phobics are statistically more likely to do so. In other words, Sam might have failed to make his peace with the unintegrated part of himself and finally been destroyed by it.

PEOPLE WHO ASK FOR HELP WITH PROBLEMS WHICH, WHILE STILL INVOLVING THOSE AROUND THEM, ARE NOT PRIMARILY TO DO WITH CURRENT MARITAL OR FAMILY RELATIONSHIPS

By now it will not be surprising to see the same themes recurring in people whose problems are not primarily to do with marital or family issues. John and Andy, for example, were both in different ways haunted by memories of their dead fathers.

John's story

John, aged 35, and his brother had watched their father, who lived with them, slowly dying over a period of three months. John's father was a proud and stubborn man who steadfastly refused to go into hospital or take his medicines, thus hastening his death and driving his sons to distraction. On one occasion John, the main caregiver, lost his temper and shouted, 'Why don't you bloody well drop dead then, if that's what you want?'. A few weeks later his father did die, and John was overcome by remorse and guilt. He could only deal with his feelings by drinking. This became too much for his girlfriend who left, taking their young daughter with her. In despair, John managed to 'arrange' his admission to a psychiatric hospital by getting into a fight and being arrested. Later he said that he had done this because he was afraid of going into a downward spiral of losing his job and getting into trouble with the police.

John had had a spell in hospital shortly after his mother's

death four years previously. The discharge note from psychiatrist to GP was along the standard lines and the diagnosis was 'inadequate personality'. This time, because of his drinking, John was diagnosed as an alcoholic and assigned to an educational programme on drinking problems. The real problem, as a proper assessment would have revealed, was unresolved bereavement coupled with the loss of his family, and his drinking had only started a few weeks earlier as a response to these events; but such subtleties are often overlooked in the routine processing of new patients.

John was surprisingly, almost compulsively cheerful in his first week in hospital. Occupational therapists reported that he never stopped rushing around from pottery class to discussion group to table tennis. Cheerfulness was not a problem to the staff, although from a psychological point of view it could be seen as yet another way to fend off grief and guilt now that he was not allowed to drink. What did concern the staff was his subsequent gradual withdrawal into misery and silence. Far from welcoming this as a sign that John had finally begun the necessary grieving process and offering him support while he went through the painful stages of mourning, John's doctors became alarmed at this turn of events. From a medical point of view, all forms of unhappiness tend to be equated with a diagnosis of depression, which is something which needs to be controlled as quickly as possible. John was therefore started on a course of anti-depressants. The irony is obvious; he had come into hospital because he knew that it was not right to try to drown his problems by taking a drug, alcohol; but as soon as he started some real work on his problems, he was prescribed another drug to suppress them again. But although John commented, 'I don't know what good these pills will do — but the doctor told me to take them', he was horrified at the idea of asking his doctor what they were for or how they were going to help.

To cut a long story short, John did eventually receive bereavement counselling from one of the staff. Although the clash of treatment approaches continued, John was eventually able to let down his defences enough to do his mourning. The climax was reached on the third anniversary of his father's death, when he sat up late into the night pouring out his guilt and despair to one of the nurses. This was a turning point for John. Nine months and much support later, he had redecorated his house, thrown out his father's clothes, and was confidently applying for new jobs. He and his girlfriend had decided to part, but he was in regular contact with his daughter. In fact for someone whose personality was now officially diagnosed as 'inadequate' he had done remarkably well for himself.

Andy's story

Andy, on the other hand, had a diagnosis of 'obsessional neurosis'. During his eight-year, on-and-off history of giddiness, depression, anxiety, and fear of dying, he had had two four-month spells in hospital and seen a succession of doctors as an out-patient in between times. In hospital, he, like Elaine and Susan, had been given behavioural treatment focusing on his symptoms. For example, he had been taken out on walks of gradually increasing length to overcome his fear of falling over with dizziness. Both in and out of hospital, a small pile of notes from psychiatrist to GP documented changes in his medication. After eight years, there were distinct signs of Persecution, which is usually conveyed in such phrases as, 'No doubt he will still complain about side-effects', or 'Unfortunately there is a histrionic flavour to his complaints'.

Eventually, Andy came to the attention of someone who was willing to help him look at his difficulties from a whole-person point of view. In accordance with the principle of over-determination of neurotic symptoms, there turned out to be several strands to Andy's problems. One of the most important was the relationship with his violent, overbearing father who had died ten years previously. The death of a relative about whom one has had intense and ambivalent feelings is the hardest of all to come to terms with, as John's story showed; but although the hospital staff had known Andy's history, they were untrained in psychotherapy and unable to put this information to use. What quickly emerged in therapy was the horrific tale of Andy's father's physical brutality to his mother, which continued right through her slow death from cancer. Moreover, Andy blamed himself for everything that had happened to his much-loved mother, believing that it was only his imminent birth that had forced his parents to marry at all.

Although Andy was by this time happily married with children of his own, the repercussions from his appalling upbringing had spread into every area of his life. His 'obsessional neurosis' apart, he carried a huge burden of guilt about being alive at all. He felt a failure as a husband and a man. Suicide seemed the only sensible option to Andy, who believed very strongly that everyone would have been better off if he had never been born. His failure to recover from his neurosis increased his sense of guilt and inadequacy, which indeed he only managed to assuage by working three times as hard as anyone else in his job at a local factory.

Like many people who have been damaged by their parents, Andy had consciously chosen an extreme opposite path to them and had resolved never to show any anger at all to his own family. Although this was obviously an improvement in some ways, it fell short of a genuine resolution to the problem, leaving Andy with no means of dealing with the anger that he inevitably sometimes felt. In particular, he had no way of expressing his anger towards his father — and the guilt he felt for his murderously intense feelings of hatred was overwhelming. Since his father's death, this had been compounded with remorse for not reciprocating the hesitant overtures that his father had occasionally made to him. Andy had been unable to cry at the funeral — another source of guilt — and had tried to block the whole of the past out of his mind. But some of his statements in therapy gave a clue to how his unconscious mind was working. He likened himself to 'a murderer who goes into court with a smile on his face even though he knows he's guilty'. After a relapse he described himself as 'a prisoner who's pulled back into jail'. At some level, Andy believed that he had killed his father with his murderous wishes, and that his symptoms were the rightful punishment, his life sentence.

The turning point was reached in a fantasy exercise. Andy had described a feeling 'as though someone's stuck a knife in my back'. Knowing that he had a strong visual imagination, his therapist asked him to close his eyes and explore this image in fantasy. Suddenly Andy was able to see who was holding the knife handle — it was his father. As his father finally withdrew the knife, Andy experienced a flood of life and warmth through his body. From that moment his symptoms receded.

A few weeks afterwards Andy was discharged and went back to work. A year later, his symptoms had not returned.

Andy, like Elaine and Susan, had had a behavioural as well as a medical approach to his problems: for example, he had been encouraged to go out on walks despite his dizziness. Behaviour therapy puts its main emphasis, as its name suggests, on changing a person's behaviour rather than on searching for deeper underlying causes. It lies at the opposite end of the spectrum from psychoanalysis, where the main emphasis is on deep-rooted issues in the past, with very little attention given to what concrete, practical changes a person can make in day-to-day life. Needless to say, both extremes miss out a good deal. Full-scale, five-times-a-week, lying-on-a-couch psychoanalysis is virtually unavailable on the NHS, and fairly difficult to obtain privately unless you are very wealthy and live near London. In the NHS, psychotherapy or counselling is much more likely to be of the sort that lies in the middle of the spectrum, like the examples we have already seen. Although all aspects of the patient's life, past and present, will be taken into consideration, the main emphasis is on change and restoring the ability to cope with everyday life rather than on acquiring insight for its own sake, so that issues will probably not be discussed in the depth that proper psychoanalysis demands. A few psychiatrists, a larger number of psychologists and social workers, and a small but increasing number of nurses and occupational therapists do this kind of work, but in many parts of the country you would be lucky to find it. As we have seen, patients commonly go through entire psychiatric careers without being offered counselling or psychotherapy. For every Elaine, Sam, or Andy who eventually reaches someone trained in these approaches, there are scores who never do.

Behaviour therapy techniques are more widely practised, probably because at their most basic they are fairly straightforward and easy to understand. Even at this level, they can be useful. For example:

A young woman cannot leave the house without shaking, sweating, and panicking. She overcomes her agoraphobia (not a fear of open spaces, but a fear of leaving a safe place) in a series of steps. With the aid of advice on how to cope with her anxiety, she gradually builds up from walking to the corner the road to going into a nearby shop, then taking a short bus ride, until she is able to travel to the town centre and spend several hours in a supermarket with only a little anxiety.

Another woman is terrified of spiders. She is helped to build up confidence by following a sequence from looking at pictures of spiders, to sitting next to a toy spider, and so on in graduated steps until she is able to tolerate a spider running over her hand.

A man is involved in compulsive checking rituals. Every day before he leaves the house he feels compelled to check and re-check the windows, sockets, fires, and switches several dozen times. At night the rituals take several hours. A nurse may be assigned to spend a day at home with him preventing him from checking. There are agreed penalties for doing it, and his family is instructed not to reply when he asks for reassurance that the lights really were turned off. He keeps a daily chart of his progress.

Behavioural techniques, then, can be very valuable at the right time and used in the right way. More sophisticated practitioners will start off with a thorough assessment of all aspects of a person's life to get a full picture of the part the symptoms are playing, and may well include counselling as part of the treatment package. The difficulty arises when staff who have no proper training in behaviour therapy or any other type of therapy and no one who is more experienced to supervise them, adopt these apparently simple techniques for any problem that comes along. Behavioural techniques may then be prescribed rather as medication usually is, i.e. without any understanding of the wider issues at stake, because staff are not trained to make this kind of assessment and have nothing else to offer. Sometimes there is a successful outcome all the same. On other occasions, as we saw in Andy's case, the problem is not solved. This is a valuable clue that more complex issues are involved and that the whole problem needs to be reassessed; but if the staff do not have the skills to do this, or even to recognize that it needs to be done, they may simply persist in the same approach even if it is not doing any good. The treatment gradually acquires a more Persecutory flavour as the patient is punished for not getting better. Thus, even after several years of an unsuccessful behavioural approach, Andy's treatment still consisted of being taken out on walks to overcome his fear of collapsing, despite his mounting desperation and his increasing conviction that he was a failure as a patient as well as in every other area of his life. A similar situation arises where behavioural techniques applied to a totally inadequate formulation of the problem ('Elaine and Susan cannot do the housework; make them do the housework') actually reinforce the dilemma that led to the problem in the first place. One of the commonest situations where behavioural language is used to justify Persecutory behaviour is when an awkward patient is defined as displaying 'attention-seeking behaviour', for which the appropriate behavioural solution is to ignore the patient thought to be trying to draw attention to themselves — known in the jargon as 'not reinforcing the undesirable behaviour'. But so-called 'attention-seeking behaviour' may be the only way a desperate or unsophisticated patient knows to ask for help. It is all too easy to use this formulation to justify not actually offering understanding or help to the least attractive and most deprived patients on the ward.

The moral is that all treatments, however simple and straight-forward they appear to be, must be applied within a whole-person, whole-system understanding of the problem if they are not to be either useless or positively harmful.

Some of the saddest stories come from young people who start their psychiatric career before they have even left their teens.

Karen's story

Nineteen-year-old Karen had a catastrophic sequence of preg-nancies, abortions, and broken relationships behind her when she was persuaded to come into hospital 'for a period of observation'. Karen had been complaining that her mind was a blank and that she could not think straight. She was terrified and panic-stricken, demanding pills and ECT to put her right, and could hardly sit still or listen to anyone for more than a few minutes. One of the doctors spent a lot of time trying to gain her trust and confidence, and slowly met with some success. After one session, Karen poured out her feelings to this doctor in a letter.

Dear Doctor X, I know what is wrong with me . . . I started blocking all my thoughts out because I could not bear thinking of what happened at the office. I met another bloke, his name was John, I probably used him to try to forget Phil but I could not. Eventually I was still blocking all of my thoughts out and thinking I was in a right muddle. I was trying to fall in love with John but could not so I just stuck with him miserably. . . . After a month I began to realize I might be pregnant. I felt so miserable I did not know what to do. I did not really want John's baby but I did not want an abortion. . . . After being five months pregnant I fell over on the pavement and lost the baby . . . I was very upset. About this time I met Alan, he started taking me out and I thought maybe this relationship would work, but it didn't. I felt as if I was going out of my mind, I was clinging to somebody all the time for comfort because I was so scared of my mind and how weak it was. Then Alan started hitting me . . .

It took another two pages to chronicle the disastrous events (including another pregnancy and an abortion) that culminated in her admission to hospital. It was hardly surprising, as Karen herself realized in her less frantic moments, that she could not seem to think straight, and her doctor spent much time patiently reiterating that no, she was not going mad, but she did need help gradually to start talking through the awful things that had happened to her.

Unfortunately, these attempts to understand Karen's difficulties in a whole person context were undermined by the message from the rest of the hospital. She was terrified at finding herself in a mental hospital along with some patients who were very disturbed. 'The other patients frightened me — I was scared of turning out like that.' Moreover, the consultant who admitted her and had overall responsibility for her case saw Karen's blank mind not as an understandable reaction to her situation but from an exclusively medical point of view as a possible sign of a schizophrenic breakdown. Karen was therefore started on medication which, as she probably discovered by comparing notes with other patients, was the same as that prescribed for the disturbed people she was so terrified by. The official medical view was, as so often happens, in marked contrast to the more down-to-earth opinions of the nurses who were actually in daily contact with Karen. One of them described her as 'just a screwed-up young girl; she's confused in her life and she doesn't want to take responsibility for anything, so she blames it all on her mind.' Nevertheless they were required to act in conformity with the medical view by keeping her in hospital and handing out her medication.

A few weeks later, the doctor who had been spending time with Karen finished her six-month placement in the hospital and had to break off the meetings and move elsewhere. Meanwhile Karen, predictably continuing her frantic search for a good relationship with a man, had picked on a young male patient who was every bit as unsuitable as her previous choices.

Perhaps it was fortunate that Karen decided to discharge herself soon afterwards. She said that some aspects of her stay had been quite enjoyable but as she also remarked, 'In here you get so much done for you, meals and tablets and things, you lose your independence. I felt there wasn't a way out, I might be in here for the rest of my life, so I discharged myself'.

Karen's story illustrates several points. One is that the demand for ECT or medication sometimes comes from patients themselves, and it is important for staff to evaluate the reasons for these demands and decide what is in the patient's long-term interests, rather than just agreeing to something which may seem the simplest short-term solution all round. Fortunately Karen's demands for ECT were recognized for what they were — another attempt to block out her horrific experiences without learning to deal with them — although the powerful medication she received instead carried the implication that her blank mind was the start of a serious illness. A much more appropriate use of medication in Karen's case would have been to prescribe mild tranquillizers on a short-term basis as part of an overall plan to reduce her anxiety enough to build up a relationship with her doctor. Unfortunately many psychiatrists work on the principle of bringing in the heavy guns first. Rather than starting with simple listening, advice, reassurance, and perhaps counselling or family meetings, falling back on physical treatments if other approaches fail, the first line of attack tends to be admission, drugs, and/or ECT.

It is not surprising that patients demonstrate inside the hospital the same patterns of behaviour as outside. Elaine continued to put on a brave face and look after others both inside and outside; Sam was passive and complaining in both places; John pushed his sad feelings away; and Karen searched desperately for a male partner. The hospital can respond in various ways.

First, and most commonly, it can ignore the behaviour, especially if it causes no inconvenience to the smooth running of the ward. Elaine's brave face went unremarked for fifteen years. Sam's passive compliance was not questioned. Thus, maladaptive ways of behaving may continue unchallenged throughout hospital treatment. Second they may be actively encouraged. It is convenient for staff and patients to have someone around like one depressed housewife who dutifully made the night drinks for the whole ward, or the forceful young businessman who rushed around organizing discussion groups and table-tennis tournaments. The fact that both these patterns of behaviour illustrated the very problems that had brought them into hospital in the first place was unappreciated. These patients were seen as helpful and co-operative, as good patients.

Third, the patient may be Persecuted, as was in danger of happening to Karen with her newly formed relationship. If she had stayed around long enough to leap from this male patient to several others, she could well have ended up being described as manipulative and attention-seeking.

Fourth, and most rarely, the behaviour can be recognized as an integral part of the patient's problems and the opportunity to do valuable work can be seized. Thus, Elaine was eventually encouraged to use her hospital stay to experiment in different ways of relating to people, without concealing her feelings or looking after others the whole time. Sam practised being assertive, while John gradually allowed himself to experience his grief. The staff missed the chance to discuss with the young businessman his driving need to take responsibility and control, or to work with Karen on her characteristic way of relating to men.

What had Karen gained from her hospital stay? She had been brought in 'for observation' two months earlier. This, or 'for assessment', is often given as a reason for admitting people. It is usually a sign that the psychiatrist does not know quite what to do with the person, who is distressed and yet falls between the categories of the obviously ill and the clearly well, but feels that something has to be done. The implication is that a skilled assessment will be carried out and a treatment plan drawn up if necessary. In fact, as in Karen's case, treatment in the form of medication is invariably started immediately and the so-called period of observation or assessment stretches into weeks and months. Moreover, since the assessment stage has in fact been omitted, neither staff nor patient have a clear idea of why this person is in hospital at all. If there are no clearly agreed goals, it is impossible for nurses and occupational therapists to know how they can help the patient while she or he is in hospital, or what are the criteria for discharge. Thus the days and weeks pass, usually until either the patient gets fed up and discharges her- or himself (as Karen did) or is discharged or transferred to another ward or hospital as a result of Persecution by the staff.

The more subtle damaging effects of a psychiatric admission, especially on someone as young as Karen, are rarely appreciated by mental health workers. To an ordinary person, coming in 'for assessment' is meaningless; the act of going into a mental hospital at all is confirmation, to them and their family and friends, that they have crossed the boundary between sanity and madness. Karen had learned to construe her understandable, if severe, difficulties in growing up as signs of abnormality. Seeing herself in this light, she is that much more likely to fall back on the psychiatric services — despite her dissatisfaction with them — in future difficulties, and to receive more of the same sort of treatment. Her family are also more likely to view her as set apart and different in some way, and to see any future problems as indications of illness or craziness. These views are shared by the wider world, employers in particular. Karen will be legally required to admit to her psychiatric history on job application forms, and this may affect her employment prospects. She will also have to disclose any psychiatric treatment on applications for driving licences, visas to travel abroad, and health insurance. Patients who have been admitted to hospital compulsorily may come up against problems with housing associations or private landlords who want information about their mental health, may find it harder to get overdrafts and loans at their bank because of an assumption that they are incapable of looking after their financial affairs, and will be more likely to lose custody of their children in divorce. There is no legal procedure to remove inaccurate statements from medical records. Even if Karen manages to overcome her problems, the long-term consequences of having a psychiatric history will stay with her for many years.

3

The sick role

After everything that has been said so far, it may come as a surprise that anyone should actually choose the career of psychiatric patient. Nevertheless there are many people who do just that and who are prepared to go to enormous lengths to find their way into hospital. Once inside, they are often the most difficult and demoralizing patients to deal with. Typically they absorb enormous amounts of staff time and energy, acquire a whole assortment of diagnoses, run through every possible treatment, are discussed at numerous case conferences, and still fail to get better.

To understand how this comes about, we need to have a closer look at what it means to be called 'mentally ill' in our culture. First, we need to remember that being admitted to psychiatric hospital is, to most people, synonymous with being mentally ill, a 'nutter' or a 'loony'. The very word hospital, with its complement of doctors, nurses, wards, and medicines, implies illness, although as we have seen most psychiatric patients are not actually ill at all.

Second, there are the powerful cultural assumptions that go along with being labelled as mentally ill. These have been summarized as:[1]

(a) You are supposed to be unable to recover by a conscious act of will. You are not responsible for your disability, and 'can't help it'.

(b) You are exempted from certain social obligations and commitments.

(c) You are supposed to see being sick as an undesirable state, and want to get well.

(d) You are seen as being in need of specialized help, which is obtainable by becoming a *patient*.

All of this applies to illness in general. Mental illness carries the additional implications that you have lost your reason, and are therefore probably unpredictable, impulsive, and liable to behave in deviant ways.

What all this adds up to is that the mentally ill person is *not responsible*. Absolute responsibility for that person therefore falls on the shoulders of the doctors. To the extent that doctors are influenced by the cultural image of mental illness, which is one of a Victim, they will be involved in taking absolute responsibility for, or Rescuing, their patients.

We have seen how this can be very destructive for people who are engaged in a genuine struggle to resolve their difficulties. However, for those who do not know how to resolve their problems, who cannot bear to face them, and have few alternative ways of obtaining care, the illness role may be the most attractive option available. We saw how it was easier for Elaine's family to push her into the sick role than to face up to their own part in her difficulties. Sometimes people in Elaine's position actively play along with this — it is easier for them, too, to accept an illness label. Sometimes they initiate the labelling process themselves by starting to act in a crazy way. Seeking help from an expert whose recommendations are to be followed obediently is a socially sanctioned way of dealing with all kinds of difficulties and distress, while the whole psychiatric set-up invites and reinforces crazy behaviour on the part of the patients.

Official entrance into the sick role is marked by receiving a doctor's diagnosis, and/or by crossing the threshold into hospital. It is, of course, possible to play the same game at a lower level by using a reputation for having 'nerves' or taking pills as a strategy. High level players aim to get admitted, because they know that in the common cultural view this is equivalent to being mentally ill. In fact they can often catch doctors out by manoeuvring admission 'for assessment' or 'for observation', and then digging their heels in and refusing to move. By this stage it is too late for the doctor to decide that, on closer assessment, they are not ill at all. They now have a psychiatric history, and can tell people they come from St X's hospital. This is more than enough to label them as ill in the eyes of the general public, and they use the public, plus agencies such as the police and casualty departments, to put pressure on doctors to readmit them.

Once inside, there are many benefits to be reaped. You can escape from painful conflicts and decisions outside. At the same time you can, if you play your cards right, gain indefinite care and asylum away from the pressures of the outside world, in a place where your bed will be made, your meals cooked, and all responsibilities lifted from you. What is referred to by mental health workers as 'the community' — i.e. everywhere that is not the hospital — often fails to live up to the cosy image that is implied. The community for many people is a bleak, lonely place of isolated bedsitters and queues in DHSS offices. In contrast, the little communities that build up in hospitals, especially on long-stay wards in the old-style asylums, can be lively and sociable worlds where everyone can find a particular role to play. There are ways of getting a good deal of attention from staff and patients; indeed, in subtle ways, you can become a very powerful figure on the ward.

It is often unclear just how consciously such roles are adopted. There is evidence that all categories of patients may have more control over their symptoms than they are given credit for.

> Bizarre behaviors present for years typically are not manifested on trips to town or when dressed up for activities such as a dance with volunteers. Within the hospital, an interview with the ward physician is a time to emit complaints and sick behavior, while less of this behavior, both verbal and motoric, is observed in 'free' situations in the ward dayroom and even less in directly productive activities such as occupational, physical and athletic activities.[2]

This is not to deny that these people are genuinely distressed — after all, such a desperate strategy implies an equally desperate problem in the first place — but to point out the inadequacy of medical model explanations of symptoms and reactions. 'Sick role' patients often end up trapped within this role and unable to break out of it even if it started off as more of a deliberate strategy. The nurses, the lowest members of the medical hierarchy, are the most likely to suspect game-playing while doctors are still juggling with treatments and diagnoses. Ultimately the only way to test out suspicions is to challenge the sick role. This is often very hard to do. But it is only by challenging the role that its hidden power is exposed, as Jeanette's story clearly shows.

Jeanette's story

Jeanette, a thin, unkempt woman who looked much older than her 43 years, had been very hard to cope with on the ward. She had good days and bad days but usually she would not get up, dress, wash, or eat without constant coaxing. She did not mix with the other patients or converse with the staff, except to say 'I don't know' or complain that the Devil was making faces at her. Her difficult behaviour included incontinence, making strange grimaces, falling over (usually outside the nurses' office) and having to be picked up, and getting into the bath with all her clothes on. Her eyes were vacant, her movements slow and shaky, and her walk was shuffling. She puzzled the doctors and frustrated the nurses.

It was difficult to piece together much information about her, but it was known that she had had an unstable upbringing as one of six children. Her first husband had been violent and her second an alcoholic. She had had various abortions, accidents, and overdoses, and only one of her four children still kept in contact with her. Now she was divorced and living on her own. Jeanette's psychiatric career had started a few years previously, around the time of her divorce. She had been admitted to several other psychiatric hospitals, nearly always after a crisis in the community. The most usual routes into hospital were via the police or the casualty department. She would refuse to answer questions except with 'I don't know' or a vacant stare. Admission 'for observation' or 'for assessment' usually followed, with a query under the heading 'Diagnosis' in the files. Over the years, the following suggestions had been made: agitated depression; obsessional and neurotic personality; schizophrenia; personality disorder; depressive illness; pseudo-psychotic. She had also been given about ten different drugs, ECT, neurological tests, and brain scans, none of which produced any improvement or threw any light on her problems.

When Jeanette moved house, she came into the catchment area of another hospital where, as described, her condition seemed to be steadily deteriorating. The familiar routine of changing drugs, ordering tests, and referring to other specialists for opinions was well under way with no obvious benefit at all.

Finally, the staff decided to take a new angle on the problems Jeanette was posing. Some of the nurses who had been involved with the tedious business of coaxing her through every step of the daily washing, dressing, and eating routine had started to suspect that she might be exploiting her status as a mentally ill patient. They decided that they had two options: to stop trying to make her better in the face of her passive resistance and transfer her to a long-stay ward, which was what she seemed to be angling for; or to challenge her sick role behaviour. They decided to challenge her role.

The plan that was drawn up was:

that a date should be set for her discharge, and she should be informed of this and asked what help she needed to prepare herself and arrange accommodation and so on;

that the staff should consistently refuse to reinforce any of Jeanette's behaviour that fitted in with the idea of being ill — for example, they should not run to pick her up off the floor, or comment on her grimaces. Conversely, they should reward her for more responsible behaviour — for example, praising her for turning up to meals.

It was predicted that if the staff suspicions were correct, Jeanette would switch from passive helplessness to active resistance in an attempt to restore the status quo. She would start behaving in a much more 'crazy' way to pressurize the staff into letting her resume the safer, more familiar role of mental patient.

Of course, it can be very hard for staff to put into action what might seem to be very heartless behaviour to a frail old lady — and Jeanette was always related to as an elderly lady, although in fact she was only in her early forties. The cultural view of mental illness which underlies nurses' training courses puts the emphasis on protecting and nursing patients, not confronting and challenging them. The distinction between being firm and Persecuting has to be made very carefully. Jeanette was not being denied help; in fact the staff were prepared to go to considerable lengths to help her find somewhere suitable outside hospital and prepare her for greater independence. What they *were* denying her, in a firm but non-Persecutory way, was the option of a career as psychiatric patient under the guise of being mentally ill.

Any doubts that the staff might initially have felt about this plan were, however, dispelled as the predictions were rapidly fulfilled, confirming their suspicions and showing Jeanette's apparent helplessness in a very different light. She began smashing plates on the ward. In accordance with the plan, Jeanette was told that she was held responsible for this behaviour, that it was not acceptable on the ward, and that if it continued she would be discharged for twenty-four hours. Jeanette continued smashing plates. A place in a hostel was arranged for her, money supplied, and a nurse was assigned to escort her to the bus stop. Jeanette's shuffling gait and shakiness had mysteriously disappeared — but as the hospital chaplain approached, she suddenly collapsed on the ground in a heap. The chaplain stepped forward to offer this distressed lady assistance, only to be told briskly by the nurse that Jeanette was quite all right and was about to catch a bus. Ten minutes later, the nurse, checking to see whether Jeanette had caught it, found that she had moved to the one stop where the bus was not due to call that afternoon. She was firmly redirected.

Meanwhile the local police, the casualty department, Jeanette's GP, and her daughter had all been warned of possible trouble and told that Jeanette was to be treated not as ill, but as fully responsible for her behaviour.

That night, the psychiatrist on duty received telephone calls at regular intervals with news of Jeanette's progress through the town. At 1 a.m. the police rang; they had been called out after Jeanette had smashed the cupboard in her hostel room. Should they bring her into hospital? They were advised not to see this behaviour as a sign that she was crazy and needed admission, but to send her away. Several other police stations through the night, ringing in to say that they had a patient from X hospital who seemed to need admission, had to be given the same advice. So did the casualty department at 5 a.m. So did Social Services at 6 a.m. At 7.30 a.m., Jeanette's daughter rang in to report that Jeanette had arrived on the doorstep saying that she had no money; she was advised to take her in only if her behaviour was reasonable. A few hours before the twenty-four-hour deadline expired, Jeanette arrived back on the ward escorted by her daughter. She was once again docile, but the power and determination behind her supposed confusion, frailty, and helplessness could no longer be doubted.

The staff had held admirably firm throughout the first skirmish, but Jeanette had not given up the fight. There were many further dramatic scenes both on and off the ward over the next few weeks. To cut a long story short, the staff held their ground and an all-round solution was reached when Jeanette accepted a place in a hostel for ex-psychiatric patients, run along family lines by a kind but very firm landlady who was not prepared to put up with any nonsense from her charges. They were expected to do their share of the chores, get out and about, mix with the other residents, and behave responsibly. There was plenty of praise when they did so and a firm telling-off if they did not. Under this common-sense regime Jeanette, the formerly fragile, helpless patient, was transformed. She became sociable, outgoing, and active. A few months later, one of the nurses was hailed in the street by a well-dressed, friendly middle-aged woman. It was Jeanette, whose shuffling gait and blank expression had vanished.

Obviously, absolute consistency and firmness on the staff's part is crucial to a successful challenge. This is rarely achieved. More often, there is a mixed approach, some staff trying to challenge the role while others reinforce it, with results like the following.

Alice's and George's story

Alice Brown, 40, was admitted to hospital with a strange series of complaints. According to her husband, George, she had been throwing herself to the ground, hitting people in the stomach, and trying to eat lumps of coal. At her assessment interview, Alice sat in a rigid posture with glazed eyes fixed on the middle distance, answering 'I don't know' to all questions in a strange, vague voice. The consultant thought that her behaviour might be due to a brain tumour, and ordered a series of tests. On the other hand it might be the sign of a psychotic breakdown, so he also prescribed the relevant drugs. In any case, he was certain that she needed to be in hospital.

One of the junior doctors, however, suspected that the underlying problem was a marital conflict. He and a nurse invited the couple to a joint session to see if they could get a clearer idea of what was going on.

George used the first half of the session to describe all the details of what he saw as his wife's mental illness. He answered all the questions addressed to his wife, insisted that she needed to be in hospital, and denied that there were any marriage problems. As the interview progressed, Alice became increasingly stiff and glassy-eyed. She professed in her strange, vague voice not to remember any of the incidents her husband described, including a recent one which involved her chasing him around the house with a broken bottle.

The doctor found himself becoming irritated with both of them. Eventually he breached all the cultural assumptions about mental illness by bluntly insisting that in his view, Alice was neither ill nor in need of hospital care, that she was quite well aware of her actions and (addressed to George) did not need George to speak for her.

The couple were both very startled. George protested, but the doctor held his ground, and gradually the whole tone of the interview changed. Alice reluctantly admitted to recalling some of the details of the chase. The nurse suggested that she had perhaps been feeling angry at the time. Alice confirmed this by producing a stream of accusations against her husband, changing as she did so from silent rigidity to furious resentment. George, though shaken, steadfastly maintained his position that he could not possibly blame his wife for irrational beliefs and behaviour that were obviously due to a mental illness. However, as the accusations continued, his annoyance became more and more apparent and soon the couple were in the middle of a blazing row ranging back over many years of accumulated grievances. The nurse commented that there was a great deal to be sorted out in the marriage, the couple were offered further meetings to help them do this, and both were sent home.

So far so good; but George and Alice were not going to be

caught out that easily. A few days later, George by-passed the junior doctor and nurse, who had agreed to be available in case of emergencies, and managed to arrange a home visit by the consultant. This, of course, was the best way for Alice to re-enter the sick role, and indeed after a few more bizarre symptoms had been described by George and demonstrated by Alice, she was readmitted for more neurological tests.

This put the junior doctor in a very difficult position. His attempts to tackle the problem at a marital level were being seriously undermined by the consultant going over his head to act in accordance with a medical model approach, and thus (in the junior doctor's view) colluding with both George's and Alice's desire to avoid facing up to their relationship difficulties. Whenever they wanted to avoid uncomfortable issues in marital counselling, they could choose an easy route into hospital again. At the same time, the doctor was very hesitant about challenging a senior colleague who had many more years of experience — and on whom, incidentally, he relied for a reference for his next job. He began to doubt his own judgement. Perhaps Alice really was ill after all, and needed a mood-stabilizing drug to put her right.

The nursing staff, too, were left in an awkward position. Nurses do not decide who should be admitted and why; they have to stand by the psychiatrist's decisions. For at least some of them, being required to treat Alice as sick and in need of medication and her husband as irrelevant to the problem conflicted with their own observations and intuitions about the situation. Nevertheless it is as rare for nurses to mount an effective challenge to a psychiatrist's medical model decisions, as it is for psychiatrists to unite in an effective challenge to a patient's sick role. Nurses are left to work out their own unsatisfactory compromises on a day-to-day basis in the demoralizing muddle of treatment approaches.

There were many more dramas over the next few weeks, involving the police (after Alice ran away from home in her nightdress), the casualty department (after she turned up there at midnight clutching an empty bottle of pills), and an assortment of Alice's and George's concerned relatives. An extremely complex history emerged of affairs, sexual problems, and family feuds, all of which had previously been invisible behind the label of a randomly occurring mental illness. A consistent treatment approach was never arrived at. If the latest crisis landed Alice at the consultant's feet — and the couple seemed to be trying to ensure that it did — then more admissions, physical investigations, and drugs were prescribed (with no improvement in Alice's mental state). The junior doctor and the nurse, meanwhile, tried hard to work on the marriage problems when the couple turned up for sessions, which they did not always do. Eventually the junior doctor's contract ended, he moved on to a different hospital, and the marital counselling was abandoned. After several more months of medical treatment something seemed to change and Alice stopped presenting herself to the psychiatric service, although no one knew quite how or why this had happened. It remains to be seen whether this apparent improvement will last.

Most commonly, however, there is little or no recognition of when or how sick roles are being exploited, and the patient follows an uninterrupted downhill path to chronic, long-stay status.

Fay's story

Fay, 63, had led a reasonably active and successful life until she was admitted to hospital, although she had always been a frequent visitor to her GP with various physical complaints. She had lived with her parents until her late thirties, but eventually married a man who took over most of the planning and decision-making for both of them. They had no children. He was nearing retirement, and she had already stopped work, when he developed an illness that was almost certain to kill him within a year. Fay became increasingly unhappy and preoccupied with physical complaints of her own. He complained that he could not cope with her at home, and, largely for this reason, a psychiatrist admitted her to hospital.

Once inside, Fay quickly took advantage of having crossed the sanity/madness threshold. On the first day, she evaded direct questions about her feelings and her husband's illness by voicing a string of complaints about backache and stiff legs; she seemed very unhappy, but was clearly-spoken, rational, and physically mobile. By the third day, nurses were reporting that she seemed to be 'picking up' some of the symptoms of the other patients on the ward. She had also started to limp. On the sixth day she refused to get out of bed, saying she could not walk. On the eighth day she refused to eat or drink. On the tenth day she told the doctor that she was mad.

To the psychiatrist, all this was confirmation of how right he had been to admit her in the first place. However, the nurses who had the day-to-day care of her insisted that she *could* walk, move, and eat perfectly adequately, but just did not want to. Referral to an orthopaedic surgeon revealed no physical cause for her limp. The nurses were left with the thankless task of trying to restore Fay to an approximation of her state on first arrival, which entailed hours of coaxing her to eat, dress, and take a few steps down the corridor, in the face of considerable passive resistance. She still refused to speak about her husband's impending death and became very agitated when the subject was raised, fending it off with renewed complaints about her aches and pains.

Fay became increasingly difficult to deal with. Sometimes she would emerge from the toilet extending hands smeared with faeces. Her husband's reaction was strange. The nurses noticed that on his visits, he would urge her to sit down, take things out of her hands, and comment on how painful walking must be for her. What was his part in the whole set-up? Since no proper joint assessment was ever made, it is impossible to say, but it certainly looked as if he too had some investment in maintaining his wife's sick-role behaviour.

Three weeks after admission, Fay presented a pathetic picture. This formerly well dressed woman sat trembling in a chair, her clothes and hair in disarray, slowly rubbing her stiff legs. Her face was closed off and vacant, and her eyes were glazed. When approached she murmured in a small shaky voice, 'I've just got worse, mentally and physically, I don't know what's going to happen to me, it's a nightmare, my legs are so stiff, my back hurts, I can't walk properly, I'm going backwards all the time'. Asked about her husband, her trembling increased. 'I'm killing him — I can't cope with his illness — I just moan at him and drive him away — I'm so selfish — it's all my fault — I feel so angry inside, I don't know why — I'm terrified of what's going to happen if he dies . . .'

Despite the best efforts of the nursing staff, Fay continued to deteriorate mentally and physically. A month later she was transferred to a long-stay ward for chronic patients in the local asylum. She will almost certainly remain there until her death, which may not be very far away.

The category that includes Jeanette, Alice, and Fay overlaps with the fourth group described at the beginning of Chapter 2, those who use the hospital mainly to meet social or economic needs. Their main problem may be that they live on their own in an isolated bedsit or a vandalized tower block, that they have no friends and little money, that they have quarrelled or lost contact with their families, that they cannot find a job, or that they need a psychiatrist's letter of recommendation to get better housing or to take early retirement on health grounds. In any of these situations the warm hospital environment with regular meals, constant cups of tea, and company whenever you want it, can be a very attractive alternative. Nor is it too difficult to gain admission by complaining of depression and suicidal impulses, which can be revived whenever discharge is threatened. Having to take medication is a small price to pay for your stay. All psychiatric hospitals develop a sub-culture of such patients, who may indeed have had a raw deal in life and be in need of assistance. The problem is that the medical model treatment they will receive along with the food, company, and so on will not solve the real practical problems that they face outside hospital. Instead it gives them the handicap of a psychiatric diagnosis and history, which will certainly not help their employment prospects or search for accommodation, while permitting them to become involved in a dishonest transaction with the staff whereby they have to trade psychiatric symptoms in exchange for shelter and company. The game is rarely challenged or exposed, although the presence of large numbers of such patients is very demoralizing for the nursing staff. On the one hand the staff are required to treat them as though they are in need of psychiatric care; on the other hand it may be obvious that their problems are not really psychiatric ones at all, and so the nurses become involved in the unsatisfactory pantomime of having to provide nursing care for patients whose real needs are for something quite different. Once again, the problem lies in the medical model approach on which traditional psychiatry is based. A model based on a greater understanding of social factors might lead to some such strategy as ensuring that they are receiving all the benefits, they are entitled to, making links with voluntary organizations and helping these people to set up and run their own clubs, support groups, and drop-in centres well away from the hospital and the psychiatric labelling that goes with it, which besides being of more help to them, would make unnecessary their entrance into the Victim position at the cost of many thousands of pounds to the NHS.

A similar problem arises for those patients who are invited to use the hospital for 'time out' (the fifth group described in Chapter 2); in other words, they simply need a rest, a break, 'asylum' in its original sense. This can be a legitimate and valuable way of using an admission, and it may be all that many people require in order to recover and get back on their feet again. But the traditional psychiatric set-up is not designed to allow for this. Anyone who comes into psychiatric hospital acquires a diagnostic label and a psychiatric history, even if their real problem is straightforward exhaustion. Patients who thought they were coming in for a rest tend to find themselves shepherded off to groups and activities along with everyone else. They will almost certainly be given some kind of medication during their stay, and factors such as noise and lack of privacy may make the hospital a very unrestful place to be.

The sixth category consists of those suffering from conditions of definitely physical origin, such as head injury, the different types of dementia (e.g. Alzheimer's disease, Pick's disease, Huntington's Chorea), and various others. It is essential to be able to identify the cases (more common in the elderly) where psychiatric symptoms turn out to be indications of an underlying organic disease. For example, memory and language impairment, visual hallucinations, and schizophrenic-type symptoms can be signs of a cerebral lesion, while brain tumours may give rise to depression, euphoria, anxiety, or irritability. Poisoning by alcohol and other drugs and chemicals, vitamin deficiencies, liver failure, and various other factors can all affect mental functioning.

The diagnosis of an underlying organic problem is often a very difficult one to make, and obviously it is essential for the psychiatric team to have access to someone with the medical expertise to carry out this kind of assessment, even if the need only arises rarely outside of work with the elderly. Whether or not it follows that only someone with medical training is competent to head the psychiatric team and make the final decisions about all types of patient, is another matter. In fact, once the diagnosis has been made (and in many cases this is best done by a psychologist using psychological tests rather than by a doctor), medical science has very little to offer to most victims of head injury or dementia, since there is no known cure. The most helpful interventions are behavioural (setting up groups to stimulate old people's memories, drawing up programmes to help with washing and dressing) and social (arranging attendance at day centres, organizing laundry services, and brief admissions to hospital to ease the burden on relatives).

The stories of Jeanette, Alice, and Fay bear all the hallmarks of people who have adopted the sick role. They had each been assigned to a bewildering variety of treatments and diagnoses, which in Jeanette's case came from several different institutions. The diagnoses varied wildly from organic (e.g. brain tumour) to functional (agitated depression) while attempts at treatment ranged from ECT (Jeanette) to marital counselling (Alice) to physiotherapy (Fay). This is in marked contrast to the other patients whose stories we have followed, who tended to get the same treatment throughout their hospital careers.

Second, they had all absorbed an enormous amount of staff time. While patients like Elaine and Susan tend to receive the most cursory discussions in the ward round ('Mrs Jones, a known depressive, was admitted again last night and has been started on X. She had a good night's sleep and has been assigned to an occupational therapy programme') many hours had been spent in fruitless debate as to how best to manage Jeanette, Alice, and Fay. Nurses had spent hours talking Jeanette and Fay through washing, dressing, and feeding, and doctors had answered many midnight emergency calls on Jeanette's and Alice's behalfs.

Third, there were the 'symptoms' which were both bizarre — eating coal, grunting, falling over, smearing faeces — and fluctuating, so that all three had periods when for no apparent reason they were rational and co-operative. These 'symptoms' did not fit clearly into any of the usual categories of mental illness — hence the difficulty in agreeing on a diagnosis.

Finally, and most interestingly, all three had begun to look and behave like long-stay psychiatric patients. Jeanette had perfected the shuffling walk and blank face of the institutionalized inmate who has spent forty years on a locked ward. Alice's speciality was rigidity and vagueness. What was so strange about this was that none of them had spent more than a few months in total in hospital — Fay had spent less than three weeks. This raises the fascinating question of how often the classic burnt-out look of long-stay patients is due to institutionalization, and how often it reflects a positive choice of a career in hospital, and a semi-deliberate adoption of behaviour in line with cultural assumptions about how crazy people act.

Obviously, you cannot ask outright to come into hospital for an indefinite period in order to escape problems outside and with no commitment to or help with confronting or resolving anything in your life. If you can find a way of entering the sick role, though, all this will be granted unto you. To do this, you need to act in such a way that other people will see you as mentally ill and take you along to a psychiatrist, so that you can maintain your position of not being responsible for what is happening. If you are married, like Alice and Fay, you can use your partners in this way, especially if they are equally keen to avoid confronting the real issues. If your problem is a lot to do with isolation and loneliness, you may need to rely more heavily on agencies such as hostel staff, casualty departments, and the police. Confronted by your Victim presentation, the psychiatrist will find it very hard not to do a Rescue and admit you.

Since mentally ill people are also seen, as we have noted, as unpredictable, violent, and irrational, you will also be able to take advantage of your status by creating all sorts of havoc without being held responsible. For example, Alice, by presenting herself as sick, was not held accountable for chasing her husband with a broken bottle. It was also easier for him to see her behaviour as craziness, rather than intense fury at him, so that he could take on the more comfortable role of concerned sympathetic husband of a sick woman.

Of course there are some disadvantages too. In keeping with the cultural assumptions about illness, you are supposed to see it as an undesirable state and to want to get well. You will be given all sorts of tests and treatments by the staff, which may be welcome in so far as they confirm your sick role. But you will also have to find a way of not benefiting from all this without arousing the suspicions of the staff. Usually, being vague and forgetful (Alice) or helpless and shaky (Jeanette) will suffice. However, if the staff apply the most effective test of the genuineness of your illness and challenge your role, your resistance will become increasingly obvious. Once the staff overcame their reservations about what initially seemed very heartless behaviour to a frail sick woman, Jeanette's strength and determination were highlighted very clearly. Even so, the patient still holds some strong cards. One resort is to approach the psychiatric system from another angle, as Alice and George did when they bypassed the junior doctor to get to the consultant. Another is to raise the stakes in the game — and this shows very clearly the enormous hidden power of the sick role, and indeed of Victim roles of any kind. Thus, Jeanette and Alice were able to create huge crises in the community, knowing that the community would place enormous pressure on the doctors to comply with the cultural image of illness, take responsibility for them, and admit them. Another powerful threat is that of suicide.

The other main disadvantage, from the patient's point of view, is that the reasons for the genuine distress which they are certainly experiencing cannot be openly expressed either because it would give the game away. This distress often has a large component of anger. It became increasingly apparent that Alice was torn with fury, jealousy, and resentment towards her husband, but presumably she could not bear to express this openly and face the conflict and the possibility of losing him. She therefore paid the penalty of having all her angry actions discounted and ignored by her husband and by most of the staff.

Jeanette's problems seemed to start around the time of her divorce, but she had to show her bitterness and anger at how life had treated her by indirect means, which still left her burdened with unresolved despair and resentment. What might be called strategic incontinence — that is, being incontinent of urine and/or faeces at times and places where it is most inconvenient for the maximum number of people — is a common device. Fay was perhaps faced with the most desperate dilemma. She felt totally unable to bear living without her husband. It was too painful to talk or even think about, and she resorted to expressing her distress in a way already familiar to her — through complaints about her physical condition. At the same time, she seemed to be overwhelmed with anger at being abandoned by him through death. But how could she express this rage to a sick man, or even fully admit it to herself? The result was terrible: she ended up driving him away even as he was dying, which only led to crippling feelings of guilt. This, at any rate, was what seemed to be going on. Looking to the future, the indications were that she would be quite unable to accept or mourn his death, but would remain paralysed by unresolved grief and anger.

From the staff point of view, these patients are extremely hard to deal with no matter what line is taken. A ward with half a dozen Jeanettes all soaking up staff time and energy without ever improving is an extremely demoralizing place to work, and the low-key but long-term effects of psychiatrists' decisions to admit such patients will be borne mostly by the nurses and occupational therapists. Although the real issues may be recognized by some of the staff, it will be impossible to get patients to do any real work on them (for example, enabling Fay to talk about her husband's impending death); because at the same time the hospital is offering a means of evading the whole problem — thus Fay no longer had to live with and witness her husband's increasing frailty, or visit him in hospital, or answer friends' enquiries about him, or plan where she would live, or face the harsh reality of the situation in any way.

Even if the role is challenged, a consistent approach may be made impossible by the ever-changing rotas and shifts of doctors, nurses, and students, to say nothing of the other patients, any one of whom might reinforce the wrong message by, for example, running to pick Jeanette up when she fell over. The psychiatric hospital is the very worst environment for someone like Jeanette who may do better in a hostel run by a single kind but firm landlady working on a basis of common sense rather than theories about mental illness.

On top of this, staff will need to be able to tolerate the very high levels of anxiety that such patients will create if challenged. In fact, the staff will be effective in direct proportion to the amount of anxiety they are able to bear. This is especially true of the psychiatrists, who will be held primarily responsible for the patient's behaviour by the community. They will need to withstand what will sometimes be intense pressure from relatives, GPs, the police, and others, who may abuse and threaten psychiatrists who refuse to adopt their counterpart of the sick role and take total responsibility for a patient. Most psychiatrists do not like being addressed in this way, particularly by their medical comrades, the GPs, whom they often go to great lengths to keep happy. It is easier all round to admit the patient and let them and the rest of the staff bear the cost.

How can these situations be avoided?

The key word is *responsibility*. The inability to take responsibility runs through all the assumptions behind the mental patient role — exemption from social obligations, being unable to help yourself, irrationality, and so on. It is central to the definition of a psychiatric patient that he or she is *not responsible*, and it follows that the hospital staff, doctors in particular, are expected to take responsibility in their place. Thus the whole Rescue game starts up.

Yet it is not enough to tell patients that they are responsible for their own problems and dismiss them, as tends to happen in Persecution. Clearly they are genuinely distressed and in need of some kind of help. What is needed is recognition that patients are responsible, capable agents, *and* in need of help as well. The one state of affairs does not contradict or cancel out the other. This means that when patients behave in a way that implies lack of responsibility they must be challenged. It also means that help must be given in a way that acknowledges a patient's responsibility for him- or herself, and his or her own life.

Let us look at how this would work in practice in the cases we have been discussing. First, attempts to force entry into the sick role, i.e. to present oneself as irresponsible and as a Victim, will need to be blocked. Such situations can readily be recognized when the patient first appears in front of the psychiatrist. Apart from the familiar hallmarks of bizarre symptoms, the involvement of other agencies, etc., the patient presents him- or herself as having no responsibility for his or her arrival or behaviour, and refuses to make a direct request for anything. At the same time the doctor feels a powerful pressure to Rescue or take responsibility for the patient. The covert request for admission needs to be blocked, and the various ways of denying responsibility (being vague, saying 'I don't know' or 'I don't remember', taking advantage of the role by hitting people or being incontinent) need to be challenged.

Second, the offer of help needs to be addressed to a whole person living within a whole system of relationships and not just to a supposed illness, so that the patient is still seen as a responsible agent. For Alice, this meant offering marital therapy. For Jeanette, it might have been an offer to find a suitable hostel or day centre where she could get support and make social contacts. For Fay, it could have been counselling to help her come to terms with her husband's impending death and plan for life on her own.

However, it is equally important that help should be offered in a way that implies the patient's responsibility for making choices about his or her life. Thus, it is no use prescribing marital therapy ('I want to see you both weekly from now on'), or a hostel place ('I'm arranging a bed for you in St John's Home') rather like an alternative form of medicine. This does not acknowledge the patient's ability and indeed right to consider the offer and perhaps refuse it. Since the patient has not played an equal part in the decision, she or he may have no commitment to the form of help offered, and may express this by missing sessions, creating scenes in the hostel, and so on. The offer, then, needs to be phrased in some such way as this:

> It seems to me, Mrs Smith, that you are wanting to be admitted to hospital. I am not willing to do that, partly because I do not see you as having a mental illness, and partly because I don't think that admission would solve your problems, which I suspect are to do with your marriage. What I am willing to offer is a series of sessions with both of you, with the aim of discovering how problems in your marriage might be contributing to your difficulties. This might be a painful task for both of you, but I believe it is the best way of helping you both in the long run. We could start with two meetings to see how things go, and then review the situation. Do you want to take up this offer?

Since it is the *way* in which help is offered that is so important, it is possible to include forms of help that otherwise tend to imply illness and helplessness (medication, admission, and so on), by doing this in such a way that the patient retains responsibility and the Rescue game is avoided. Thus, instead of 'I am prescribing you' (or, addressed to a relative, 'her'), 'some pills to take three times a day', or 'I think you/she had better come into hospital for a while', the psychiatrist might ask the patient if she or he wants medication or admission. This forces the patient to make an explicit request and thus take a share of responsibility for what happens. This request can then form the basis for negotiation between the two parties, perhaps along the lines of:

> I want to make it clear that I do not see you as having a mental illness. However I would be willing to prescribe you a sleeping tablet/tranquillizer to tide you over this crisis. Some people get a dry mouth or slight headache as side-effects, so you should tell me if that happens, but they are not addictive if

taken for a few days only. Do you want to have some?

Or:

Although I don't see you as being ill, you are certainly in a difficult situation at the moment. If you wanted to come into hospital simply for a break and a rest, I would be willing to offer you a bed for three days. But if you are going to solve your problems in the long run, I believe you will need some counselling help as well. Do you want to be admitted on this basis?

The differences in approach might seem small, but they are crucially important. If the Smiths, or whoever, accept the offer of counselling, then a major — perhaps *the* major — piece of work has been done. They will have shifted their attitude from blaming everything on an illness suffered by one person, to acknowledging emotional problems in both, and the psychiatrist will have gained their active commitment to working on these problems.

If, on the other hand, the Smiths refuse, then at least the whole destructive, time-consuming Rescue game has been avoided. Depending on how hard a game the couple are playing, Mrs Smith may put up resistance by acting crazy, and the psychiatrist will need to stand his ground. Or the Smiths may try and get into the psychiatric system some other way, or try another agency.

Probably there will be some middle course. Several crises may have to be dealt with along these lines before the Smiths are ready to take up the offer. At difficult points in the therapy they may switch back into the Rescue game, as Alice and George did. Again, the psychiatrist and the team will need to stand very firm.

In summary, a *treatment contract*, based on *mutual consent*, needs to be drawn up and agreed between both parties. Doctors often claim that patients have consented to treatment. However, mutual consent involves a great deal more than the patient saying 'All right then' or 'I'll try anything' when a doctor recommends medication or admission. As in legal contracts, mutual consent implies that the patient has made an explicit request for help with a clearly defined problem; that the doctor has made an equally explicit offer of a clearly described and understood form of help; that the patient understands the contribution he or she will be expected to make to treatment; and that he or she has accepted the offer.[3] In this way, the people who use the psychiatric services can turn from patients — a word which implies the sick role, a passive waiting on expert advice — into clients, consumers who are actively selecting and participating in their own treatment.

But all this does not just apply to people like Jeanette, Fay, and Alice. It applies to *all* patients. We saw how the Rescue Game operated so destructively in the stories of Elaine, Susan, Sam, John, Andy, and Karen, so that they were either pitied/Rescued/seen as 'mad' or blamed/Persecuted/seen as 'bad'. The whole Rescue Game can be avoided by drawing up a proper treatment contract based on equality, mutual consent, and a whole-person, whole-system understanding of the situation.

When Elaine was first referred to a psychiatrist, an elementary knowledge of psychology should have been enough to recognize the very common pattern of breakdown in a woman who is trying to give to others when she has never been given to herself. Although a full understanding of the problem was only reached after several months' counselling, Elaine's breakdown could have been explained in simple terms to her and her husband after the first interview as the delayed effect of her emotionally deprived childhood coupled with current stresses in the family. This would have set the framework for the treatment contract. Elaine might still have been offered (not ordered) admission and/or medication, but with the clearly explained aim of rest and recovery from the present crisis so that the underlying issues could be tackled. Such a contract would have given the nurses and occupational therapists the necessary guidance to make their contribution to the treatment plan, perhaps helping her to choose relaxing activities instead of cooking, and encouraging her to take care of herself for a change. In the longer term, counselling sessions could have been offered to Elaine. The scene would also have been set for involving Elaine's husband and perhaps her whole family at some point. Fifteen years before the entrenched situation that we saw in the first chapter, Elaine and her husband might have accepted this explanation and offer with relief and understanding. There is every reason to suppose that Elaine would have responded as constructively as she did fifteen years later. Her husband might well have learned to make use of counselling too, with the probable result that his own difficulties would have become an equally important focus of treatment. And with luck, many of the destructive patterns that later emerged in their children would have been avoided.

Andy, on the other hand, probably never needed admission or medication at all. Again, an elementary knowledge of psychology should have been enough to guess at a connection between his appalling relationship with his father and his subsequent dizziness and fears, to suggest to him that this was worth exploring, and to offer him a treatment contract of outpatient sessions to do that.

John, who was dealing with his grief by drinking, already realized quite clearly that he needed help over his father's death. What he had trouble with was framing his request for help. He arranged his admission by getting into a fight rather than by asking openly for what he needed. The psychiatrist responded by doing a Rescue, admitting him to hospital without an agreed contract and moreover with a mistaken idea of what the basic problem really was (bereavement, not alcoholism). John's first interview should have been spent clarifying what he was asking for and negotiating over what could be offered. This would have made the staff's role clearer, if he had been offered admission after all; he did not need talks on the evils of drink, or distraction with lots of activities. Instead, he needed people to be with him and gently encourage him to start the process of mourning.

It is vitally important that treatment contract negotiations start from a person's very first contact with the psychiatric services. The initial interview is of absolutely crucial importance. If the first meeting ends in a Rescue rather than a negotiated contract, if one person out of a system is labelled as the sick one, or if all the difficulties are attributed to an illness, then the whole direction of treatment has been set. Staff, patients, and relatives will take up their positions accordingly, and it may be extraordinarily difficult to frame the problem in any other way at a later date.

Let us illustrate these points by accounts of two initial interviews.

Mr Harris's story

Mr Harris was sent up to the psychiatric hospital by his GP as an emergency referral, with a letter saying that he had cut his wrists after a family row, was a suicide risk, and needed to be admitted.

Mr Harris was practically incoherent when he was seen. He slumped in the corner of the psychiatrist's office sobbing and shaking, apparently unable to say anything except 'I don't know why I did it, I just want to end it all'. There were two shallow scratchmarks on his wrists.

Mrs Harris was asked in and gave a clearer account. The couple had been celebrating their twenty-fifth wedding anniversary with a large party two nights before. At some point during the proceedings, Mrs Harris had discovered her husband embracing one of the female guests in the hallway. It was not clear to what extent this was simply a friendly gesture on his part, but Mrs Harris had certainly not taken it that way. She had stopped the party, created a huge scene, and threatened to leave him. Their teenage daughter had apparently already moved out in disgust at her father's behaviour, while Mr Harris had been weeping and threatening to kill himself. Mrs Harris angrily told the psychiatrist, 'He must be sick to behave like that! You're the expert — you've got to make him stop. He must be sick or the GP wouldn't have sent him up here!'

It would have been very easy to yield to the open demands from Mrs Harris and the GP, and the less explicit but more powerful pressure of Mr Harris's helplessness, and arrange for him to be admitted then and there. But instead of being pushed into this course of action, the psychiatrist wanted to find out what lay behind this strange story. He told Mrs Harris firmly that her husband was upset but not sick, and asked what had been so very distressing to her about the incident at the party. As she filled in some of the background, Mrs Harris became less angry. There were long-standing marital and family problems, and Mr Harris's role seemed to be that of whipping-boy, with his wife and daughter forming an alliance against him. Mrs Harris had in fact had an affair herself a few years ago. It began to look as if the party incident had been an excuse for each side to get back at the other. Mr Harris could repay his wife for her affair by being discovered in a situation that was bound to provoke her, whereupon she flared up and threatened to leave him. He then raised the stakes and threatened to kill himself, and she turned angrily on him declaring he must be sick. He went along with this, Persecuting her by his fearful helplessness and implicitly asking the psychiatrist to Rescue him. This the psychiatrist refused to do. The discussion had helped Mrs Harris reach the point where she could admit that she had been at fault too. She was even prepared to retract her threat of leaving her husband. Mr Harris was still tearful, but the psychiatrist judged that his superficial scratches were more of an attempt to cause alarm than to take his life. He therefore took the calculated risk of dismissing them both with a joint appointment to discuss their disagreements in more depth the next day. By that time the crisis had blown over, and it was even possible to do some useful work to prevent a similar situation recurring.

If Mr Harris had been admitted, the family view of him as the sick, weak one would have been confirmed, making it very difficult if not impossible for other hospital staff to introduce an alternative approach. This is the position that nursing staff often find themselves in. The crucial admission work is done by psychiatrists, and the person who arrives on the ward has already been selected out of a network of relationships as the sick one, and given a diagnosis of illness.

Mrs Moore's first interview was not handled so well.

Mrs Moore's story

Mrs Moore was a 55-year-old widow whose elder daughter reported to the GP that she was losing her memory, accusing other people of hiding things round the house, and doing a variety of other strange things. In a brief interview, Mrs Moore did seem unhappy. The psychiatrist accepted her daughter's selection of Mrs Moore as the sick one in the family, and persuaded her to come to hospital as a day patient. Mrs Moore did not really want to do this, but bowed to the combined pressure of GP, psychiatrist, and elder daughter. After a few days she stopped attending although her daughter's complaints were becoming more frequent. The psychiatrist sent a social worker to visit the house and see if Mrs Moore needed compulsory admission.

Here, a very different scene presented itself. Mrs Moore explained apologetically that she really did not want or need to come into hospital. Nor did she like the idea of taking pills. She had certainly been feeling very harrassed recently, because of rushing around trying to please everyone in the family, but she was starting to sort things out on her own. Mrs Moore's elder daughter was out, but the younger one was at home. Hardly had the social worker started to ask her for her view of the situation when she burst into tears, and he found himself trying to help a completely different member of the family than the supposed patient. This daughter explained that she felt desperately torn between life with her husband and their two children a hundred miles away, and looking after her mother. Mother had seemed to be doing fine until the elder daughter rang up with all kinds of dreadful stories about her, and even threatened to have her put away in psychiatric hospital if she (the younger daughter) did not come down at once and take a turn in looking after her. It emerged that there was a long-standing battle between the two sisters, and mother's supposedly strange behaviour (for which no concrete evidence was ever found) was being used as a weapon in the latest fight. The social worker spent some time encouraging the younger daughter to assert herself and decide how she wanted to live her life. He also encouraged the mother to make her own decision about whether she wanted professional help. Mother and daughter were both greatly relieved, and nothing further was heard from the family.

The absence of proper treatment contract negotiations makes it alarmingly easy for relatives to arrange for someone to be admitted, for good reasons and not-so-good ones. A proper first interview would have established that Mrs Moore did not want or need hospital care. What she might have welcomed help with was standing up to those who thought they knew best for her — including the doctors.

It may be thought very strange that these dangerous muddles routinely occur in psychiatry, and that in many places it is virtually unheard of for a patient to be asked such simple questions as, 'Why are you here? What do you want help with? How will we know when you are better? When do you want to leave?' But to do so challenges the whole medical model on which traditional psychiatry is based. People who are sent to general hospitals with physical complaints are not expected to work out for themselves what the cause is, nor are they asked to decide what kind of treatment they want — these are questions for the doctors and nurses. Psychiatry as a branch of general medicine is based upon the same principles, and the training that psychiatric staff receive makes it extremely difficult for them to view it in any other way.

In the next chapter I will consider whether the treatment contract approach has anything to offer to people who are out of touch with reality or, in simple terms, mad, and who might seem to be the most suitable candidates for medical-style Rescuing.

4

The treatment barrier

WHERE FAMILY RELATIONSHIPS ARE SO INTENSE AND ENTANGLED THAT ONE PERSON IN THE SYSTEM BREAKS DOWN VERY SEVERELY

Jenny's story

Jenny Clark was a 20-year-old student of hairdressing, living at home with her parents. Her brother, several years older, had left home to marry and her younger sister was away at teacher-training college.

Unlike her more outgoing brother and sister, Jenny had never had many friends of either sex. She found it very hard to talk to people, and at school had sometimes been teased for her slight stammer when she was nervous. She did not seem to be settling in very well at college either. Most evenings and week-ends were spent at home, despite the rather tense atmosphere there. Her mother had been brought up in a deeply religious Catholic family in a small town in Ireland. She had met her English husband, her first boyfriend, when she was a shy and inexperienced 19-year-old, and moved to England with him. Over the years the couple became disenchanted with each other, and ended up living almost as strangers in the same house. With the failure of her marriage, Mrs Clark's children became even more important to her. She only spoke of her husband with bitterness and resentment, and he withdrew into himself and became the butt of family jokes. Neither of them had friends locally, and he spent his time either at work or out fishing while she kept the house in immaculate order.

During her second year at college, Jenny started to retreat into herself even more. Quiet and obedient all her life, Jenny had never caused her parents any trouble. Her brother and sister had been the ones who got into rows about staying out late and not helping around the house. Jenny's mother often said that she lived only for her children, and since she saw many of her own attitudes and characteristics in Jenny, they had been particularly close. Now, though, there were clashes between them for the first time when Jenny flouted various family rules and cut herself off from the activities she and her mother used to do together. She stopped talking to her parents, refused to answer the telephone, and sometimes did not go into college. Mrs Clark couldn't understand why Jenny locked herself away in her room for hours listening to records. As the weeks passed, she became more and more concerned. She even began to fear that Jenny was going out of her mind. In the end, she called in the family GP.

The GP thought that Jenny was very confused and unhappy rather than mentally ill. Jenny sat staring miserably at the floor while the GP, who fortunately had a good relationship with her, tried to coax a few words out of her. Slowly and hesitantly, Jenny opened up. Her whole life was a hopeless failure, she said. She had never fitted in at school. The other girls ridiculed her, and none of the boys ever asked her out. She had hoped college would be different, but it was turning out to be even worse. Everyone had got their little groups of friends and she was left on the outside. Anyway, no boy would ever want to go out with someone who had such big hips and freckly skin. She wasn't even sure if she wanted to do hairdressing anyway, but what else could she do? It was all her parents' fault. No wonder she had no friends when they never mixed with anyone and had such old-fashioned ideas. Living at home in that atmosphere was enough to make anyone miserable. If only they would try to understand her, but her mother just interfered and her father was worse than useless. No, she didn't want to move out — she just wanted to be able to live happily with them. Her secret ambition, she confided, was to be a glamorous film star. She had been practising expressions and poses in front of the mirror in her room.

All this information was pieced together over several sessions. Jenny, driven in her mother's car since she refused to go out on her own, was being seen by the GP for twenty minutes or so after surgery once a week. The GP saw her as struggling with many common adolescent problems about finding her own place with her contemporaries, planning her life, and separating from her parents, and he encouraged her to start reversing her retreat from the world. Jenny gradually became more at ease with the doctor and took a few tentative steps — ordering some books for college was one, and telephoning a girl she had been at school with was another. She still clung to the idea of being a film star, despite a complete lack of acting ability or experience, and she refused to contemplate leaving home to share a flat. The whole idea of boyfriends and sexual relationships was terrifying to her. Nevertheless, progress was being made. After confiding many bitter memories of being teased and ridiculed at school, she discussed with the GP how she could handle such situations differently. One day there was a breakthrough. Jenny came to the surgery on her own, by bus. She had drawn out some of her savings and bought herself a new, fashionable pair of boots. She was going to the cinema with a girlfriend that weekend, and was more cheerful and confident than the GP had ever seen her. He told her how delighted he was, and privately anticipated tailing off their meetings.

This was not to be. The next evening, he received a frantic telephone call from Mrs Clark, who said that Jenny was refusing to come down to meals, and she was sure her daughter must be going crazy. The GP dismissed this idea, advised Mrs Clark to leave Jenny's food in the oven for her, and promised to bring the subject up with Jenny the following week. Mrs Clark did not seem at all reassured. The next day there was a similar telephone call. Mrs Clark insisted that Jenny hadn't eaten for two days, that she was pacing round the house muttering to herself in a crazy way, and that she needed to see a psychiatrist. The GP agreed to call round that evening. The atmosphere was extremely tense. There was no sign of the strange behaviour that Mrs Clark had reported, but Jenny was more openly angry with her mother than he had ever seen her. She furiously accused her of forcing her to eat fattening food when she was trying to diet, and of generally treating her like a baby. Mrs Clark yelled back that anyone who could say such things must be crazy — Jenny had never behaved like that before — she must be ill. The GP tried in vain to help them reach some kind of compromise, but feelings were running too high. He withdrew, telling them they would have to sort this one out themselves, to which Mrs Clark retorted that he was useless at his job, and anyone could see that Jenny was ill.

It was the on-call GP who received the next telephone call later that evening. By the time she went round, Jenny was extremely agitated and unable to sit still for a second. As the GP opened the door, Jenny seized her coat and rattled off a long speech about how much she hated both her parents, how her mother had suffocated her all her life and never let her grow up, and how everyone treated her like an idiot. This was interspersed with such strange remarks as, 'I can fly out of here any time I want, you know. I know the GP is really married to me. I know everything'. Simultaneously Mrs Clark tried to engage the GP's attention by yelling her version of events — that Jenny was crazy and dangerous and needed to be taken away, just as she'd been trying to tell people for months. A furious screaming match broke out as Jenny shook her fists and let rip with pent-up resentments against her mother — 'I hate you! You just want to keep me like a child! You never leave me alone!' while her mother retaliated at the top of her voice with 'You're crazy! You're mad! You should be locked away!'. As the accumulated family tensions of many years exploded round his head, Mr Clark hovered ineffectually in the background, wringing his hands and remonstrating feebly with both of them.

The GP felt totally out of her depth, and also alarmed at some of Jenny's bizarre remarks. She decided that the best thing to do was to call in the psychiatrist and the duty social worker. When these two people arrived at the house, they accepted Mrs Clark's word that Jenny was violent, and agreed that she was also deluded, a danger to herself, and in need of hospital treatment. Forms were signed for Jenny's compulsory admission, and an ambulance was called. Struggling desperately and shouting that she was sane, Jenny was physically forced into the ambulance and taken to the admission ward of the local psychiatric hospital, here she refused to submit to a medical examination, telling the doctor angrily, 'I'm perfectly sane. I don't need to be in hospital'. She was injected with a powerful tranquillizing drug, and put to bed.

The next morning, Jenny was stunned, scared, and bewildered. One of the nurses came to talk to her as she sat dazed and silent on her bed. There was no sign of the furious struggle of the previous night, nor did she make any bizarre remarks. Instead she was trying to make sense of the catastrophic event that had befallen her. She asked anxiously, 'Does being in here mean I'm mad?'. She refused to see her parents when they visited, saying she hated them. Later in the day her dazed bewilderment was replaced by open distress and agitation. She refused her medication, accusing the staff of trying to drive her mad, and so she was held down and injected instead.

Over the next few days, Jenny slowly lost her hold on reality. Partly due to the side effects of the large dosage of drugs, the bright young woman was transformed into a shuffling creature with slurred speech and vacant eyes, a trace of saliva escaping from her half-open mouth. Despite the heavy sedative effect she kept constantly on the move, up and down the ward, muttering under her breath and intermittently pulling up her nightdress to show the nurses her supposedly too-large hips. From time to time she had outbursts which could perhaps have been seen as a frantic protest against her situation, but were interpreted by the staff as further evidence that she was sick and needed to be controlled. Thus, when she threw food and plates around, tried to escape from the ward, swore at the doctors, slammed doors, and hurled herself to the floor, more medication was produced to sedate her, in spite of her frantic cries of 'I don't want that stuff! You're just trying to slow me down!'. At other times, it seemed as though her previous worries were all appearing in a distorted form. For instance, she told the staff that Prince Charming had spoken to her from the television and was going to visit her that night. She announced that she was a film star and then that she was pregnant. Once she asked anxiously if she had killed her family, and then told one of the doctors, 'I'm only three years old.'

The Clarks, who visited nightly, were desperately upset to see their daughter in this state. When Jenny agreed to see her, Mrs Clark put her hair in ribbons and fed her sweets, though the visits sometimes ended with Jenny swearing and shouting at her mother.

After several weeks, Jenny was judged to have improved — that is, although far from her previous self, she was more often bemused and passive than furious and resistant. She was allowed home on leave, where she was visited by a community nurse. He found that Mr Clark had once again retreated into the background, while Mrs Clark's entire time was devoted to caring for her daughter. Jenny was constantly exhorted to brush her hair nicely, to eat up her food like a good girl, to sit quietly in her chair, and so on. Jenny made feeble protests at some of these instructions, but at the same time seemed unable to let her mother out of her sight, trailing after her from room to room asking 'I'm a good girl aren't I? You're not cross with me are you?'. Mrs Clark became openly furious at any suggestion that it would be helpful to encourage Jenny to be a little more independent. As far as she was concerned, the doctors were entirely to blame for not listening when she first thought Jenny was going crazy. As for Jenny, she looked terrified at the suggestion that she might one day want to go out into the world again and perhaps have a job and friends of her own. 'No, no' she said, quickly retreating into her fantasy world. She picked up one of the pictures of film stars which littered her bedroom floor and wandered round the room, saying in the childlike voice that had now become habitual, 'I want to look like her. I want to be like her'.

We will leave Jenny there. There are several possible outcomes for her and others who, like her, are diagnosed as schizophrenic. (Schizophrenia refers not to a split personality, but to a state where a person loses hold on reality and may suffer from delusions and hallucinations.) She may make a good recovery after one breakdown, as about one-half of sufferers do, and resume a normal life. She may go on to have repeated breakdowns and admissions, spending more time in hospital than out of it, as happens to about a quarter of people. Or some kind of compromise situation may be reached whereby she manages to stay out of hospital most of the time, but settles for a limited existence at home, friendless and partnerless, never quite able to break away from her family to establish independence and an identity of her own.

A number of factors seem to have contributed to Jenny's breakdown. Always more sensitive and introverted than her brother and sister, she had found it especially hard to overcome the disadvantages of an upbringing in a socially isolated and conflict-ridden family. All the same, she had the usual desires of young women her age for friends, boyfriends, and an attractive appearance. It was not very surprising that she lapsed into despair at achieving none of these, although in retrospect her very unrealistic ambition to be a film star might have sounded a warning note. However, the interesting fact is that the crisis blew up just when everything seemed to be going better at last.

Jenny was more closely identified with her mother than the other two children, and hence had a more intense and complex relationship with her. Out of the three children who had come to mean everything to Mrs Clark after the failure of her marriage, only Jenny was still at home. It was at the point when real separation became an issue, when Jenny seemed to be about to grow away from her anxious, obedient child self and her family and step into the outside world, that Mrs Clark's genuine concern over her daughter's unhappiness seemed to be replaced by a more desperate fear that Jenny might abandon her. In the commonest (though not universal) pattern, the first schizophrenic breakdown is precipitated by the threatened separation of a child from a parent (usually the mother). Hence, first breakdowns occur most frequently between the ages of 17 and 25, when young people are involved in the struggle to establish their identity and separateness from their families. If the patient is married, the issues are often the same — the struggle to achieve psychological separation from the parents, and sometimes the marital partner too, although the prognosis is usually better in such cases, since the fact that marriage has taken place means that some degree of separation has already been achieved.

Of course, separation causes conflicts and arguments in most families, but in some the struggle takes on a particularly intense quality. Typically the child or young adult has been unusually unseparated up until this point. Like Jenny, he or she is often described in such terms as 'good as gold', 'never a moment's trouble', 'couldn't bear to be apart from us', and this is seen by the parents as normal and desirable rather than worryingly lacking in the protests and disagreements by which healthy children start to establish themselves as separate individuals. If the bond is between opposite-sex pairs (mother and son, or more rarely father and daughter) the relationship may have strong sexual overtones. Sharing bedrooms or beds until a very late age sometimes happens.

After many years of 'good' behaviour, there typically follows a stage where the child, rather belatedly, starts to act in a manner that is seen as 'bad' — getting angry, answering back, disobeying rules, and so on. Most parents are able to bear this period of estrangement until the transition from a child-parent to a more adult-adult relationship is achieved, but if a parent's whole identity and life is bound up in the child, then the prospect of challenge and separation may be intolerable. The 'bad' behaviour constitutes an unbearable threat which has to be seen as beyond the bounds of reason; crazy; mad. The 'bad to mad' route by which people end up in hospital was seen in embryonic form in such cases as the Harrises and George and Alice (Chapter 3). It is the counterpart of the 'mad to bad' route by which patients get pushed out of hospital again. By labelling 'bad' behaviour as crazy, the message that the parent cannot bear to hear can be discounted. Thus the Clarks did not have to consider whether there was any truth in Jenny's accusations about them. As Jenny became more independent, the threat to the family set-up increased. So, rather than welcoming Jenny's progress, Mrs Clark became more and more terrified and her accusations of craziness escalated. Most first admissions for schizophrenia occur not as the result of a considered decision to seek psychiatric help, but during a huge crisis when life-long tensions erupt in a terrifying maelstrom. The parental or family view and the child's view become polarized as each side is involved in a desperate struggle for self-preservation. Either Jenny's (extreme) view of her mother's possessiveness and her father's uselessness will win, and the family will be forced to face up to the element of truth in these accusations, with catastrophic results for the present family set-up; or her mother's equally extreme view, that Jenny is simply mad, will prevail, with equally catastrophic results for Jenny.

At this crucial crisis point, the psychiatric services are called in. From an outsider's point of view, there is perhaps not much distinction to be made between Jenny's behaviour and her mother's. Each was screaming equally unpleasant things at the other ('I hate you!' versus 'You should be locked away!'). However, for reasons that will be discussed more fully later, the psychiatric staff almost invariably take the parental/family side. Thus it was Jenny and not her mother who was described as verbally aggressive, violent and a danger to herself. (No actual evidence of violence to another person was ever produced, either in or out of hospital, but it is a frequent accusation from relatives, and is almost always taken at face value by the professionals without investigation.) The crisis is over when the professionals yield to the considerable pressure to designate the nominated member of the family as the crazy one, and have confirmed this status by the ritual of diagnosis, admission, and medication. Whatever craziness there is in the family has then been officially located in one member, and the rest can breathe a sigh of relief. The child, however, will have been defeated in this crucial battle to assert identity and independence, probably for ever.

Once the line has been drawn between the mad and the sane, all future remarks and behaviour will be classified accordingly. Thus, the account that appears under 'Previous history' in the medical notes will probably be derived entirely from the parents and will be treated as the true version of events. A typical example might read: 'Mother dates the patient's illness back two years when she changed from being quiet and well-behaved to being aggressive, resistant, and rude. Parents have managed this as best they could until stress over exams triggered the present breakdown'. Here, the delayed emergence of normal adolescent behaviour is described, and accepted, as illness, with the final breakdown attributed to some external event. Meanwhile, the patient's point of view is discounted, because, after all, the patient is mad. At best, it might appear under the heading 'Sample of patient's speech', where Jenny was recorded as saying, 'I am all right. I don't need any medical examination. I don't know why people are making a fuss of me'. Such statements are noted for diagnostic purposes only, and their meaning is ignored.

The catastrophic effect on a sensitive young woman like Jenny of finding yourself compulsorily detained in a psychiatric hospital, feeling abandoned and betrayed by your family, can hardly be over-estimated. Your sanity depends on being able to make some sense of this appalling event — but the powerful drugs that Jenny was immediately given made it very hard for her to think this through. She was very aware of the numerous cues that told her she was deemed to have crossed the threshold into madness: the hospital surroundings, the doctors and nurses, and more subtle cues such as the tone of voice used to address her. However, her cries of 'You're trying to drive me mad!' were either discounted or taken as further evidence of madness. Some of the nurses privately thought there was some truth in her complaints about her parents, but they saw their main job as nursing a sick young woman through her illness. They had only the parental version of the events leading up to her admission to go on and were not trained to intervene in family conflicts, so they did not share their reactions with her. When Jenny did lose her hold on reality, they were even less able to make sense of her strange statements about Prince Charming, being pregnant, killing her family, and being three years old. Such remarks were simply recorded in the notes as 'delusional thinking'. Looked at from another angle, Jenny's desire to find the man of her dreams, her fear of the consequences of sexual relationships, her terror of losing contact with her family, and her acknowledgement of her childlike state, can all be recognized in these statements. Most of us speak in metaphors: 'I wish I could meet my Prince Charming', or, 'I could murder my family'. Some people who break down take the process a stage further and start living their metaphors instead. However, doctors and nurses are not trained to understand or decode such messages, and thus it was Jenny and not the psychiatric staff who earned the comment in the medical notes, 'Has no insight. Does not understand what is said to her'.

The hospital environment reinforces all of a person's most childlike aspects, which is particularly damaging for someone like Jenny whose very problem centres around the struggle to grow up and achieve adulthood. Thus she had to go to bed and get up at specified times, ask permission to have a bath, stay in her nightgown, and comply with various other ward regulations. In a tragic repetition of the situation in her family, her rebellion against these rules, against taking her drugs and against the very fact of her containment, was seen not as healthy assertiveness or understandable protest but as further evidence of her illness. The more she struggled, the more entangled she became.

But it would be very misleading to describe Jenny simply as the helpless victim of her family. At the home visit after her discharge, the symbiotic nature of the relationship with her mother was very clear. Neither could separate from the other. If Mrs Clark was terrified of Jenny abandoning her, Jenny was equally terrified of being abandoned. The unhappy result whereby each was tied to the other was a way for each of them to avoid their deepest fears. In retrospect this pattern could be traced back to before the breakdown. If Mrs Clark had not been able to promote Jenny's independence, Jenny had never been willing seriously to consider the possibility of leaving her. The fantasy of being a film star had never involved moving away from home.

It would be equally mistaken to doubt the Clarks' genuine care and concern for their daughter. Mrs Clark's reactions and behaviour were the result of her desperate attempts at a solution to her own impossible dilemmas. The departure of her daughter would threaten her psychological survival and leave her facing the emptiness of her marriage and life. The position of Mrs Clark, and of the shadowy figure of Mr Clark on the edge of the family, will be considered in further chapters.

This analysis of the experience of a girl diagnosed as schizophrenic and her family is an extremely contentious one. The same events might be described from a medical point of view along the following lines:

> This young woman showed a pattern of increasing withdrawal typical of the early stages of schizophrenia. When she became floridly psychotic, compulsory admission to hospital was necessary and the appropriate medication was given. After a few weeks she was sufficiently improved for discharge. Her progress will be monitored closely, and it is likely that she will need to take medication for some time.

While there is often informal recognition of the relevance of family relationships, reflected in such comments from the nurses as, 'she/he is fine as long as mother/father isn't around', or 'I think we've got the wrong one in here', the orthodox psychiatric view is that schizophrenia has a genetic biochemical cause, the cure for which will ultimately be revealed by medical research. Anything else going on in the patient's life is described under some such general heading as 'environmental stress' which merely acts as a trigger for the underlying illness. Alternative views are either completely ignored, or discounted, with some such textbook assertion as 'family relationships have *not* been shown to be relevant'.

In fact this is misleading. In a thorough investigation of the relevant research, two eminent professors of psychiatry, exponents of the traditional viewpoint, summarized the findings as follows:

> In our view the following statements are reasonably supported by the experimental evidence:
> 1. More parents of schizophrenics are psychiatrically disturbed than parents of normal children, and more of the mothers are 'schizoid'.

2. There is a link between 'allusive thinking' in schizophrenics and their parents, but this is also true of normal people, in whom it occurs less frequently.

3. The parents of schizophrenics show more conflict and disharmony than the parents of other psychiatric patients.

4. The pre-schizophrenic child more frequently manifests physical ill health or mild disability early in life than the normal child.

5. Mothers of schizophrenics show more concern and protectiveness than mothers of normals, both in the current situation and in their attitudes to the children before they fell ill.

6. The work of Wynne and Singer strongly suggests that parents of schizophrenics communicate abnormally, but their most definitive findings have not been replicated.

7. Schizophrenics involved in intense relationships with their relatives or spouses are more likely to relapse than those whose relationships are less intense.[1]

What they resolutely refuse to concede is that such factors contribute to schizophrenic breakdown in the first place, as opposed to being the *result* of having an abnormal child in the family, or triggering second, third, and fourth breakdowns once the first has occurred.

Meanwhile, the fact that, as one textbook admits, 'no convincing evidence has been found'[2] for a biochemical cause does not incline psychiatrists to dismiss these theories in the same way. Indeed, the reverse is true; textbooks devote many pages to such theories, while the genetic/biochemical view is generally presented to patients and relatives as a fact rather than an unconfirmed hypothesis. Thus, we have the strange situation where schizophrenia is treated as an illness with a physical cause although none has ever been discovered. This, of course, is a status it shares with almost every other condition treated by psychiatry, since only a very small minority (e.g. senile dementia, Huntington's Chorea, Korsakoff's syndrome) have a known physical cause.

The debate about schizophrenia has already attracted more than its fair share of professional and public attention. The bread-and-butter of psychiatry is not schizophrenia, but the more routine procession of depressed housewives, rootless young men, and lonely old people. More interesting and more useful than theoretical debate is a look at the remarkable and exciting approaches that some pioneers have developed by breaking away from the medical model. However, in any debate that has raged so long, so angrily, and so inconclusively there must be other issues and interests at stake. I would like to look at some of these and make some suggestions as to why the search for a physical cause of schizophrenia has become the Holy Grail of psychiatry.

Firstly, there is great pressure from the relatives of people who have been diagnosed schizophrenic to find not only a cause, but a physical cause. The anger of those who have felt blamed by a misleading interpretation of schizophrenia, 'It's all the fault of the wicked parents', is understandable. In fact, the parents are genuinely concerned people struggling with their own often very difficult lives and circumstances, and looking after the patient with minimal advice or support from the psychiatric services. This often places a very heavy burden on them. Studies show that the mental health of about one-half to three-quarters of close relatives suffers under the strain of looking after a mentally disturbed family member, while family life, household routines, social and leisure activities are all severely disrupted.[3] Blame is not a useful response to any patient or relative, whatever the problem. It is also illogical; after all parents are themselves partly the result of *their* parents' attitudes, and so on in an infinite regression. Similarly, families are themselves shaped by the often very powerful and destructive pressures of the wider society of which they are a part, a point which will be discussed further in Chapter 11. Nevertheless if relatives do play a crucial part, however unwittingly, in the development of schizophrenia, then it is misleading, unhelpful, and ultimately unethical for psychiatry to claim to be offering treatment without addressing these issues, whether the problem is schizophrenia, depression, agoraphobia, or whatever. The failure to do so is another example of psychiatry's preference for what might be called 'being kind to be cruel' — avoiding awkward evidence and scenes in the short-term while the long-term cost is borne by relatives, patients, and junior members of staff. Meanwhile virtually the only form of treatment on offer is powerful medication, which has unpleasant and often dangerous side-effects, and at best helps the patient to keep going rather than curing the underlying problem. But we shall see that the alternative approach of venturing into the lives of these families demands a great deal from the professionals; more, often, than they are prepared or able to give.

There are other vested interests at stake in the debate about schizophrenia. What is at issue for the psychiatrists is the whole basis of their claim that a medical training and approach is essential and fundamental. Until now, there have been no successful challenges to their absolute domination of the field of mental health. The debate about the physical causes of mental problems is the battleground on which the powerful medical lobby is fighting to preserve its interests. The new moves towards community care have intensified the struggles. Hospitals are being run down, and the community mental health centres that are appearing in their place may be headed by nurses, psychologists, or social workers. New counselling approaches are gaining a foothold and proving to be very effective with many neurotic patients. It is increasingly important for psychiatrists to maintain that psychotic (out-of-touch with reality) patients like Jenny are suffering from a physical biochemical disorder that only doctors are qualified to treat properly.

The philosophy of community care has led to a spate of protests from the general public. They do not want people whose dress, speech, and behaviour may breach social norms in *their* street. Articles and TV programmes have emphasized the dangerous nature of people diagnosed as schizophrenic, and called for funds for scientific research into the physical cause. It is easier for the whole community, as well as particular families, to reject the messages that these patients convey, to argue that their problems are purely physical in origin, and to campaign for them to be shut away until medical research has revealed the cure.

The drug companies also have a powerful interest in promoting the view of schizophrenia as a physical illness. They make millions of pounds a year from the profits of medication, and sponsor hundreds of research programmes. There is no financial incentive for them to promote alternative views of schizophrenia.

Many people come along to psychiatrists hoping that an easily curable physical cause can be found for their distressing symptoms. Often they are searching for a 'magic pill' to take their 'nerves' away, so that they do not have to face up to what may be painful underlying conflicts. Unfortunately, 'magic pill' answers always fail, the effects of ECT or the new tranquillizer fade, and the search starts up again. Schizophrenia is one of the most distressing symptoms of psychiatry's inability to offer real help to unhappy people, and psychiatry can be seen as desperately searching for a 'magic pill' answer which will take away the problem while validating the medical model approach on which traditional psychiatry is based. Such answers have been discovered regularly for the last twenty years, hailed as breakthroughs, and with equal regularity have failed. It seems very unlikely that a true solution will be found before there is an honest facing up to the power games and the social and political interests and conflicts that underlie the whole issue of the causes of schizophrenia.

Quite apart from all this, there are overwhelming difficulties for research to contend with. These have been extensively argued elsewhere,[4] but the main points (which apply equally strongly to other supposedly physically caused psychiatric problems such as endogenous depression, that is, depression for which psychiatrists cannot identify an obvious external cause) can be summarized as follows:

1. The term schizophrenia has itself never been satisfactorily defined. In fact it refers to a group of disorders with very different manifestations, so that two people diagnosed as schizophrenic may have no symptoms in common. Since there are no physical tests for schizophrenia, diagnosis is based on reports by the sufferer and the relatives, observations of behaviour, and the doctor's clinical judgement. This means that in practice there is wide variation in the way the diagnosis is used. In Russia, the same symptoms are far more likely to be called schizophrenia than in the UK. In some hospitals almost every other patient will be called schizophrenic, and it is difficult to avoid the impression that the term is used as a rag-bag for patients who are hard to classify. Thus, people who show none of what are called first rank symptoms (e.g. delusions and hallucinations) but are simply withdrawn, apathetic, or confused (for which of course there are many possible reasons) may receive the label. Karen (Chapter 2) is a case in point. Other psychiatrists develop their own idiosyncratic diagnostic systems, so that one doctor may prefer some such portmanteau term as 'schizo-affective disorder' while another apparently sees a lot of people with 'schizophrenia, paranoid type' or 'schizoid personality disorder'.

2. Even were a watertight definition to be agreed on, it is far from clear what would qualify as proof of a physiological

cause of the condition. We are, of course, bodies as well as minds, and it is in a sense inevitable that our physical selves are involved in schizophrenia, as in other forms of emotional distress, in some way: 'That there *are* biochemical differences in schizophrenia is certain — just as certain as that there are biochemical correlates in the brain to rage, anxiety, and learning Spanish',[5] but the fact that the two things occur together does not necessarily mean that there is a causal connection. Even if there is, perhaps it is the mental state that causes the physical one, in the same way as anxiety causes sweating and shaking. Or perhaps some third factor is involved, as when the presence of certain metabolites in some schizophrenic patients was shown to be due to the excessive tea and coffee drinking that is a part of institutional life.

There *is* evidence that a genetic factor is involved in schizophrenia, since relatives of people diagnosed as schizophrenic have an increased risk of developing the condition themselves. Recent research suggests that certain chromosomal abnormalities can be found in some sufferers from schizophrenia, although not all sufferers show the same abnormality, and, conversely, not everyone with the abnormality develops schizophrenia. The most popular current theory argues that the inherited abnormality is a tendency to overactivity in certain nerve cells in the brain which use a chemical called dopamine to transmit messages from one cell to another. However, the evidence also shows very clearly that the genetic factor is not enough to result in schizophrenia on its own. One possibility is that the genetic component is something akin to a general emotional sensitivity, which in different circumstances, as one study suggests, can manifest itself in other ways — as unusual creativity, for example.[6] Such a characteristic is not something that it is either possible or desirable to eliminate.

Almost certainly, there will be no simple 'magic pill' solution to the problem of schizophrenia; the complete picture, for this and other psychiatric problems, will involve a number of factors all of which contribute to the final outcome. Thus, inherited vulnerability, birth trauma, family interactions, social stresses, and wider political and economic factors such as unemployment and poor housing will all add a layer to the problem and increase the likelihood of breakdown in a particular individual. The question then becomes: at what level, or levels, can we most usefully and effectively intervene? At present, only the genetic/biochemical factors are being addressed by medical research which, for political rather than logical or therapeutic reasons, is attempting to find the whole answer in what can be, at best, only one layer of the problem and a very remote one at that, if indeed it is a causal factor at all. Meanwhile, despite some textbook acknowledgement of the relevance of psychological and social factors, the only treatment on offer in day-to-day psychiatric practice, for schizophrenia as for other psychiatric problems, is ECT or medication with poorly understood actions and effects.

3. Let us suppose, though, that all the above issues were to be fully acknowledged and taken into account by psychiatrists. Even this would not be enough — for what any medical approach, even a more enlightened one, crucially fails to address itself to is the *meaning* of these factors in the individual's life. For a full answer to the question of why this particular person, in this family, develops these particular symptoms at this particular time, it is not enough to add some such term as 'family discord' or 'environmental stress' or 'loss of job' to the formulation of the problem. This is no better than recording in the notes that the patient is making 'delusional remarks' with no attempt actually to understand what the patient is trying to express. Useful as the scientific/ medical approach can be, it can only take us part of the way. It cannot, for example, tell us what Jenny's failure at college meant to her, or enlighten us as to the nature of the emotional struggle between her and her mother, or decode the messages behind her strange remarks, although for anyone who had been prepared to listen, the whole story of Jenny's tragedy was encapsulated in her 'delusional statements'. But such messages are hard to listen to, for professionals as well as for families. One psychiatrist who has worked with these patients for many years believes that 'the biochemical research still being financed in the field of "schizophrenia" may well be the symbol of our obstinate attempts to *deny that human distress and confusion can take this form.*'[7]

I would like to look briefly at three different approaches to schizophrenia. The first is an example of what might be called an enlightened medical model approach and is widely recognized by mainstream psychiatrists. The other two are alternative approaches, one carried out within the psychiatric system and one outside it, which share two important characteristics. First, they have a view of schizophrenia as part of a whole person in a whole system of relationships, not just as a disease entity. The second and not unrelated point is that they have been completely ignored by orthodox psychiatry.

A well known psychiatrist, Professor Leff, and his colleagues have carried out thorough and much-quoted work with people diagnosed as schizophrenic and their families.[8] (This follows on from earlier studies by Brown et al.[9]) They rated patients' relatives on a number of scales such as hostility, over-involvement, and critical comments, and found that about half the families scored highly on these measures. This was referred to as High Expressed Emotion or High EE, while the other families were characterized by Low Expressed Emotion or Low EE. They found that the likelihood of relapse after a first schizophrenic breakdown was greatly increased if a patient lived with a High EE family. Leff and his colleagues therefore put together a package of educational talks, groups for relatives, and family sessions to try and reduce the level of EE and hence the rate of relapse in these families. The approach was a commonsense, practical one in which the professionals tried to help patients and relatives to reduce the amount of time they spent together, to build up separate social lives, to deal with arguments around the house, and so on. All the families succeeded in reducing the level of EE or at least spending less time together, and this significantly reduced the rate of relapse in the patients especially if medication (which presumably also helped to block out the effects of High EE) was taken as well. Interestingly, though, over-involvement — which included such factors as over-protectiveness, excessive self-sacrifice, the inability to lead separate lives — hardly changed at all. Meanwhile a comparison group received standard NHS treatment, i.e. no help or advice for the relatives, and the relapse rate was much higher.

Leff's work has been widely accepted in psychiatric circles (although despite this lip-service I have yet to meet a psychiatric team that actually puts it into practice), partly because it is thorough and useful, and partly because it allows psychiatrists to avoid the whole controversial issue of what led to the initial breakdown, concentrating instead on how relapse can be prevented once the first breakdown has occurred. It stops just short of challenging the medical model approach, although at one point, it seems, all this High EE might, in fact, be contributing to the whole problem in the first place.

Evidence exists linking one emotional attitude we found to be influential, with maternal overprotectiveness antedating the onset of schizophrenia . . . overprotective attitudes were more commonly shown by mothers of children who later developed schizophrenia than mothers of control children . . . This suggests that the overprotective degree of involvement develops very early in the child's life, and indeed we have anecdotal evidence of this from several of our families.[10]

One of his co-workers has written:

Separation is always the big issue . . . for some families it was possible to work towards hostel placement, in others the intensity of closeness was so great that the focus had to be on small issues. In one family, for example, months of work was spent on helping a mother and daughter negotiate the daughter's washday.[11]

Some of the thumbnail sketches of the families involved in the study confirm how blinkered it is to treat one member of the family as ill while ignoring what is going on around them. Thus:

The patient, a man of 23 living with mother, stepfather, and a younger brother, suffered a first attack of schizophrenia. Mother had always seen him as the weaker of her two sons and appeared to have been overinvolved with him virtually from birth. He slept in her bed till the age of fifteen. . . .

The patient, a woman of 24, lived with her parents and siblings. Both parents were highly critical of her, particularly her father . . . She returned home. After a few days her father had a furious row with her and ordered her to sleep in a shed in the garden. Several days later she suffered a return of auditory hallucinations.[12]

However, these clues have not been followed up. Leff's more recent work has involved attaching electrodes to the fingers of his schizophrenic patients, to measure changes in their skin conductance levels when relatives direct all this High EE at them.[13] It could be argued that this is one way to investigate innate physiological sensitivity in these patients; but this line of research can also be said not to address the whole thorny issue of the significance and meaning of these family interactions. What exactly was all this High EE about? Why did the relatives react in these ways? How did the patients feel in the face of critical or hostile remarks? What were they all saying and doing to each other, and why? None of these questions was addressed. We are left with the standard psychiatric position, that abnormalities in the families, however extreme and long-established, are the result of, and not a contribution to, having an abnormal child in the family.

Dr R. D. Scott, a former NHS psychiatrist, spent many years working with those who are diagnosed schizophrenic and their families. In contrast to Leff, he is particularly concerned with the whole process of how someone comes to be labelled as schizophrenic and admitted to hospital in the first instance, and the events that lead up to this crucial moment. His stance is very different from the orthodox one, but his findings will not come as a surprise to readers who have followed the arguments of this book so far.

Scott punctures the myth that it is psychiatrists who diagnose schizophrenia and other psychiatric problems.[14] In almost every case, he points out, the diagnosis has already been made by ordinary lay people who have selected one member of the group or family as the sick one. These lay people then put the psychiatrist under enormous pressure to rubberstamp this diagnosis while at the same time insisting that it is *he* who is making the diagnosis and not they. ('You're the expert, doctor. He must be ill or he wouldn't be here.') But if as the 'expert' he refuses to go along with this diagnosis, and refuses to say what they have told him to say, then the situation may become very tense and threatening. We saw how Mrs Clark had decided that Jenny was crazy at a very early stage, was furious with the GP who refused to go along with this diagnosis when the crisis blew up, and eventually found a doctor who was willing to do so. Similarly, Mrs Harris (Chapter 3) had already decided that her husband was sick, brought him along to the hospital to have this diagnosis confirmed, and was angry when the doctor disagreed. However, there was less at stake for her, and she was eventually prepared to alter her stance and admit her part in the problem.

Scott sees the purpose of this manoeuvre as 'avoiding mutual and unbearable pain between two or more family members',[15] which threatens to come to the fore during a crisis point in the family's life. If the doctor complies with the relatives' expectations and agrees to label one person as mad and take total responsibility for him or her, then

he will be forced to draw a line which rigidly divides the ill from the well; human relationships are then maintained in a severed and disconnected state. The parents deny that forms of relationship threatening to themselves are relationships; they are seen as forms of disturbance in the patient. Thus, symptomatology is maintained by the conventional approach whilst relationship issues are depersonalized and evaded.[16]

Scott calls this event, the drawing of the sick/well line, 'closure', and notes that 'the point at which inner disturbance in the family, which may have been present for years or even generations, becomes officially located as being disturbance in one member . . . brings relief from uncertainty — now they know what the trouble is'. At the same time, 'the cost is frightful. What happens may result in the permanent . . . crippling of one or more lives.'[17] After closure has occurred, there is an impenetrable barrier to dealing with the issues in the relationships between the patient and others. Scott calls this the 'treatment barrier'.

The operation of the treatment barrier can be detected in the other cases we have seen; it was very hard for Elaine or her therapist, for example, to untangle the relevant relationship difficulties since all the problems had been officially located in her 'illness'. What seems to distinguish those diagnosed as schizophrenic and their families from other patients is the intensity with which the dramas are played out, and the rigid finality of closure when it occurs.

A further result of the treatment barrier is that the identified patients, even if genuinely needy, can at the same time exploit their sick-role status rather as Jeanette, Fay, and Alice did. Scott again:

In our experience the power of the role . . . of mental patient is tremendous. It is a power which patients freely use: many times our patients have presented themselves at a police station, 'I'm from Napsbury'. They want a free ride back . . . I might tell the police officer, 'It is very kind of you to offer transport, but I think it would be better to let him increase his self-reliance by finding his own way back'. The chances are that the patient still arrives by police car, or else the patient may phone a relative who gets on to me and accuses me of negligence and cruelty. It is practically impossible to let a patient be responsible, and they know it.[18]

He also presents evidence that although patients are seen by their parents as fitting the cultural image of mental illness, that is, as being confused and unable to take responsibility, the patients often see themselves as controlling, while also being aware that others do not see them as possessing this power.[19] This is added confirmation of the secret power of the Victim role.

So, how can closure and the creation of the treatment barrier be avoided? Or, to put the same question a slightly different way, how can one avoid this particular variation of the Rescue game? With people called schizophrenic the question is, if anything, even more crucial than with other patients, since closure is even more final and absolute. The answer, though, is the same. Essentially, it is to resist the pressure to treat the identified patient as the helpless Victim of a disease process; to refuse to collude with hiding the relationship issues under the label of an illness; and to negotiate a proper treatment contract rather than taking complete responsibility for the patient and the 'illness'.

Scott has shown that all this is possible even with those patients who are most out of touch with reality, and apparently most suitable candidates for a medical model-style Rescue. He and his team started to do

something we had never dared to do before: challenge the role of the mental patient. At the group meeting in the admission ward we, as a team, would not take the medical counterpart of the mental patient role, but instead adopt an approach in which we might say to a patient, 'You must want something from us since you do not leave. If you could tell us about this we might be able to help'. We do not accept denials of agency, and we remain unresponsive to psychotic (i.e. crazy) types of explanation. In this way psychotic ideas can sometimes be undercut in one session revealing more real issues, the hurts, despair, conflict with others.[20]

Similarly, relatives were asked why the children came into hospital with an equally firm refusal to accept that it was entirely the result of a doctor's decision. This simple policy led to a drastic reduction in psychotic behaviour, length of admissions, and use of sedative drugs on the wards, but not without cost to the staff. 'The use of the approach has required staff to withstand a high degree of anxiety. It cannot be used by individual staff members, but requires a team organized from top to bottom.' The case of George and Alice, where only one unsupported doctor and nurse were prepared to challenge the mental patient role, illustrates this point. Again, Scott warns that breaking these unwritten rules meant that 'relatives, and patients too, have tried threatening us with the highest authorities'.

It became obvious that if this approach was to work properly, not only for people diagnosed schizophrenic but for all types of patient, then the psychiatric team would need to organize itself in a radically different way. Usually, there are a number of different routes into hospital (via casualty, the police, GPs). The person designated as the sick one will probably be seen at the hospital so that it is impossible to get a true picture of the home and family situation, or else admissions will be arranged over the telephone without the doctor seeing the prospective patient at all. If a short home visit is made, it is merely to rubberstamp the diagnosis that, as we have seen, will already have been made by relatives, neighbours, and other lay people.

Scott and his colleagues realized that there had to be a cohesive admission team prepared to travel out to homes, hostels, bedsits, or wherever the problem was and spend as much time as was needed to get a proper picture of the whole situation and every individual's part in it. Since at the start of the new approach 90 per cent of their admissions were by crisis, the team had to be available twenty-four hours a day, seven days a week, so that the confusions created by having several routes into hospital were avoided. The staff also had to be readily available for some weeks or months after the initial crisis visit, to do follow-up work and give advice and support as necessary. The crisis intervention team consisted of a psychiatrist and a social worker, and it guaranteed to be on the doorstep within two hours of receiving a call from a GP, the police, or more rarely, members of the public. The team believed that the first contact with the psychiatric services was crucial, and could determine the whole future pattern of events. A crisis was not an unfortunate event that had to be defused as quickly as possible by removing the supposedly sick person; rather, it was a unique opportunity to do vital therapeutic work, as tensions that might have been dormant and hidden for years erupted into the open. But if this chance was not seized and used, closure would occur and the conflicts would be sealed off, perhaps forever, as one member of the family embarked on the career of mental patient.

On a crisis visit, the first task was to reduce the tension and build up a complete picture of the background to the crisis. Then some sort of mutual understanding and agreement as to what was going on had to be reached. If this turned out to be a marital or family issue, then the focus would shift to marital or family counselling, perhaps followed up with further meetings over the next few weeks. Whatever the outcome, the same therapist would be involved throughout to co-ordinate the treatment. If one person was admitted to hospital, then great care was taken to ensure that this was not done in such a way that one person was labelled as the 'sick one' with all responsibility for him or her being handed over to the doctors. For example, there was the case of a woman who became depressed when her marriage broke up:

Her husband, to spare himself pain and guilt, regarded her as mentally ill; he blamed the marital rift on illness and persuaded her to see the doctor. The GP involved the psychiatric team because the woman's parents with whom she was living were keeping a suicide watch over her. She was seen with her parents in their home. At interview it became clear that both the parents and the woman herself were in favour of her becoming a psychiatric patient in order to punish the husband who was blamed for making her ill. After the tension had been reduced it became clear that she was not really ill, and the family found a more reasonable way of dealing with the situation, one which involved all, including the GP, in decisions and actions. The danger was that the broken bonds of feeling with her husband would become seen and used as forms of illness, and that she would become cut off as a psychiatric invalid, from which condition she might never emerge to become capable of relating to another man.[21]

In Jenny's case the team would have needed to sit with the family until the immediate uproar died down, rather than defusing the situation by certifying one member and forcibly removing her. When a measure of calm had been achieved, they would have started piecing together the events leading up to the crisis, this time taking Jenny's viewpoint into account as well. They would have tried to build up a full picture of the background: Jenny's difficulties at school, the Clarks' unhappy marriage, the role the other children played in the family, Mr and Mrs Clark's own background, and so on. This might well take several hours, rather than the half-hour or so that would be needed for a quick decision to admit one member. They would have worked towards a mutually agreed view of the problem as something in which the whole family was involved, so that even if admission had still been necessary, the way would have been open for more work on the family issues. Family meetings might have been arranged regularly for the next few months, while the hospital staff would have been informed about the background and encouraged Jenny to talk about her feelings and frustrations instead of just medicating her. In other words, there would have been a proper treatment contract, rather than a Rescue.

Leaving the sheltered world of the hospital was an eye-opening experience for the team. Scott and his staff realized that following normal psychiatric practice had meant that

> we hardly knew anything about the lives of our patients and their families. . . . We have discovered things that amazed us. We began to find out about life and it was not always pleasant. But at least it was preferable to that awful sense of arrested life that goes with closure.[22]

The team had anticipated resistance to the new approach, and in fact there was what Scott described as a 'bloody revolution' within the hospital, which found its very existence threatened by the dramatic fall in admissions. The climax of the struggle was an inquiry into the medical and nursing practices on some of the wards, which put the continuing existence of the crisis intervention team and its philosophy under threat. The team survived, but the rigidity of the nursing hierarchy meant that nurses could never be part of it.

The new approach demanded much from the staff. Scott speaks of

> the distress all members experienced when brought face to face with the realities of human relationships. When the presenting 'madness' is penetrated and the anguish and desperation is laid bare, it takes a strong stomach to continue with one's endeavour. . . . Roles tend to become blurred in the dust and murk of the coal face and the release of emotion that is often encountered is no respecter of status or discipline.[23]

Truly, it is safer and easier to stay in the hospital with the old routine of medication and admission.

Over a period of several years the number of sudden emergency calls dropped, and, perhaps because GPs had been educated to look for underlying issues, people were more likely to come along asking for help with relationship problems than with mental illnesses. More recently, closer links with voluntary agencies and other resources and a greater awareness of the effects of sex roles have influenced the way the service operates.

The crisis service still exists, although to what extent it operates as a true crisis intervention team depends very much on the attitudes of the current consultant and his/her staff; obviously it is possible to be visiting homes and meeting relatives and yet still be doing the same diagnosis-prescription-and-admission routine as before when you get there. A study of one of the original teams over a two-year period showed that admission rates were halved, with first admissions being reduced by up to 60 per cent. The resulting reduction in the number of beds enabled several wards to be closed with a saving of several hundred thousand pounds of NHS money a year.[24] American studies of crisis intervention services confirm that they are very much cheaper to run, while follow-up shows that patients do at least as well under this system as those who receive the more traditional approach.[25] Less tangibly, the new approach was felt by Scott's team to be vastly more productive and satisfying than the old one. However, it does present a strong challenge to orthodox medical model psychiatry; indeed Scott came up against active suppression from official bodies when he tried to give lectures and submit articles on his work. This is perhaps why, despite its many therapeutic and financial advantages, more than fifteen years on it has yet to be adopted by any other hospital in Britain.

The Transactional Analysis (TA) approach to schizophrenia was developed in America in the 1960s by therapists working outside the psychiatric system, who belong to what has come to be referred to as the Cathexis School. Unlike some of the other new therapies like gestalt, co-counselling, psychodrama, and so on, which seem to work best with the group of people sometimes referred to as the 'worried well', TA has also addressed itself to more serious conditions like manic-depression and alcoholism. Its basic assumption, in contrast to the traditional psychiatric view, is that such conditions can be cured, not just controlled. 'Schizophrenia is considered a solvable problem.'[26] Although TA therapists believe that there may be relevant genetic factors and admit to failure with some patients, they also claim dramatic success with their non-medical approach to some of the most seriously disturbed and damaged people, who are able to take up a normal everyday life and even to become therapists to other disturbed patients in their turn.

According to TA theory, people can operate in one of three different ego states at any one time. The Parent ego state is made up of advice, rules, values, traditions, and 'shoulds' and 'oughts' as well as permissions, encouragement, and protections derived from the person's actual parents and other authority figures. The internalized negative aspects of the Parent are sometimes experienced as messages inside the head: 'Don't make such a fool of yourself', 'You're bound to fail at this', and so on. In schizophrenia, such Parental messages may be heard literally as real voices from outside the person, in other words as auditory hallucinations. The Adult is rather like a computer which gathers and processes information about the world, and thinks it through rationally and without emotion. The Child is the source of joy, fear, anger, sadness, excitement, and so on, and of spontaneity, sexuality, and creativity.

Essentially, TA therapists, and in particular the Cathexis School, see schizophrenia as the result of contradictory messages from the Parent ego state which the Child learns to adapt to at a very early age in order to survive, although in the long term this prevents the individual from getting his or her own needs met or adjusting to society generally. In non-psychotic individuals, the Adult is able to bring information from an external reality to bear on such problems, but in people diagnosed as schizophrenic there is not enough consistency between the internal and external worlds for them to be able to do this, and they retreat into their maladaptive inner frame of reference. The Parent messages can be summed up as, 'You are not OK. The world is a bad place. My needs come first'. The Child adapts to these messages by learning that 'I am not OK. I am scared (of the world). Parents come first'. The Adult is misinformed or uninformed.

The Cathexis School aims to provide a safe and secure environment where the patient can regress back to the period before the problem began — younger than one year old. The patients do this by withdrawing energy from their Parent ego state — this is known as de-cathecting their Parent and is something which apparently only schizophrenic patients are able to do. Having discarded their Parent ego state altogether, they think, feel, and behave like children again and grow up through the various developmental stages at the rate of about one year every 6 to 12 weeks. During this time they are looked after by a therapist who has previously made a contract with them to act as their new parent, an agreement which is lifelong, the therapist being addressed as mother or father and treating the client exactly like a natural child. (This can be confusing to an outsider, particularly if the 'parent' is in fact younger in age than his or her 'child'.) The re-parenting process is a carefully programmed and commonsense one: 'Basic to our general structure is an assumption that there is an objective reality, which people can observe and mutually define. We believe it is impossible to teach people how to live without giving them value-oriented definitions by which to live.'[27]

In the early days, regression took place in a supportive setting similar to an ordinary family house where the 'parents' were available twenty-four hours a day. Now, people are treated on a day-patient basis, returning to hostels or sheltered accommodation at night. Less disturbed patients can be dealt with on an outpatient basis by making a contract with them to regress for a certain number of hours a week. 'Chronological age becomes irrelevant, and frequently it seems almost that we are running a nursery school for oversized toddlers.' In the very early stages, adult bodily functions may be lost and nappies and feeding bottles are used. It is necessary to impart the useful Parental instructions that have been jettisoned along with the damaging ones — for example, 'You should brush your teeth twice a day'. Other Parental messages, which replace the original ones and are reinforced kindly but firmly, are 'You are responsible for what you say and do', 'Feelings are OK', 'You can solve problems',

'You are expected to think', and so on. Whereas in traditional psychotherapy the aim might be to change specific Parental messages (e.g. 'You should never get angry', 'You'll always be a loser') the aim of re-parenting is for the patient to incorporate a whole new Parent ego state from the new mother or father. Issues are not dealt with in the traditional psychotherapeutic way (for example, to a persistently late client, 'Who else did you want to keep waiting when you were young?') but within the relationship, ('You're my son and I want you to be here on time'), followed by examining the issues that such a confrontation raises.

Obviously this radically different approach is very challenging to the medical view of schizophrenia, and in America it initially met with strong resistance. The pioneers of what is called the Cathexis School found that their mail was being tampered with and that they were being tailed by strange cars, and this culminated in a series of police charges initiated as a result of pressure from the medical establishment.[28] The therapists fought back and won their cases, and over time their approach has come to be recognized in the TA community. There are also therapists working with schizophrenia along TA/Cathexis lines in Holland and the approach has been used in India, but it is virtually unknown in Britain outside the TA community, although a project has recently been set up in Birmingham.

Very little research has been published on outcome, although I understand that a long-term study is being conducted in Holland. TA is oriented more towards therapy than research, and I can only say that on meeting some formerly very disturbed and now re-parented ex-schizophrenic people they impressed me not only as being free from any signs of psychosis, but also as being exceptionally capable, mature, and self-confident individuals. However, whatever its achievements, it seems unlikely that mainstream British psychiatry will extend a warm welcome to an approach that challenges so many of its basic assumptions.

5

Women's role problems and psychiatry

Women psychiatric patients outnumber men by 7 to 5.[1] Many of the problems that bring them into contact with the psychiatric services — depression, anorexia nervosa, bulimia nervosa, agoraphobia — are mostly or almost exclusively found in women. A closer look at the roles women are expected to fulfil in our culture is necessary to understand why this is so.

Let us backtrack a little and look again at the 'depressed housewife' who is perhaps the commonest recipient of psychiatric treatment. We saw in the first chapter how Elaine's depression was treated as something separate from her family, her upbringing, and her life and role as a woman. Her dilemma, unravelled in therapy, went something like this:

She had adopted the traditional woman's role of wife and mother.
She had devoted her whole life to giving to others.
Her own needs were not fulfilled.
She believed it was selfish to have anything for herself.
She could not ask for what she needed.
She resented not getting what she needed.
She could not express her resentment and felt she had no right to protest about her situation.
She broke down through giving out far more than she received.
She blamed the whole situation on herself.

In a much quoted study, Pauline Bart[2] traced these and similar themes in over 500 American women aged between 40 and 59 who had come into hospital for the first time with a diagnosis of depression. Theories have been put forward suggesting that the increase in depression in woman around this age is due to the hormonal changes of the menopause or other biological factors. A special diagnosis has been coined for the problem, 'involutional melancholia'. Bart, though, wanted to try and understand the problem from the point of view of women's role expectations. She talked to women whose breakdown had occurred shortly after a child had left home or got engaged or married and discussed what this had meant to the mothers. She found that the women in her survey saw their most important role in life as mothers and homemakers, and that they had thrown themselves into these roles with a completeness that left very little time for themselves or a life outside the family. Typically, they might say:

> I was such an energetic woman. I had a big house, and I had my family. I took a lot of pride in my cooking and in my home. And very, very clean — I think almost fanatic.

Being deprived of this role by the departure of their children was devastating:

> It's a very lonely life, and this is when I became ill, and I think I'm facing problems now that I did not face before because I was so involved especially having a sick child at home. I didn't think of myself at all. I was just someone that was there to take care of the needs of my family, my husband and children.

Previously, if these women had felt low,

> I would get up and I knew that there was so much dependent on me, and I didn't want my daughter to become depressed about it or neurotic in any way which could have easily happened because I had been that way. . . . It's just recently that I couldn't pull myself out of it. I think that if I was needed maybe I would have, but I feel that there's really no one that needs me now.

Now, as another of the women said,

> I don't feel liked. I don't feel that I'm wanted. I don't feel at

101

all that I'm wanted. I just feel like nothing. I don't feel anybody cares, and nobody's interested, and they don't care
whether I do feel good or I don't feel good. I'm pretty useless.

These women had nothing to do, nowhere to go, and no
source of confidence or self-esteem apart from the bitter
memory of having been such devoted mothers. Often, there was
a sense of betrayal and of resentment against the departed
children. This could not be openly acknowledged and was
turned inwards into despair.

I felt that I trusted and they — they took advantage of me.
I'm very sincere, but I wasn't wise. I loved, and loved strongly
and trusted, but I wasn't wise. I — I deserved something, but I
thought if I give it to others, they'll give it to me. How could
they be different, but you see, those things hurt me very
deeply and when I had to feel that I don't want to be alone,
and I'm going to be alone, and my children will go their way
and get married — of which I'm wishing for it and then I'll
still be alone, and I got more and more alone.

The loneliness was accentuated by the fact that dissatisfac-
tions in their marriages could no longer be hidden behind relentless activity. 'My whole life was that because I had no life with
my husband, the children should make me happy . . . but it
never worked out.'

The irony is, as Bart points out, that these women arrived in
their position by doing what was expected of them by their
families, their friends, the media, and society in general. To an
even greater degree than some of their contemporaries, they had
embraced the traditional female destiny of finding fulfilment
solely through being wives and mothers. But because identity,
purpose, and self-esteem were all dependent on having others
around to care for, they were empty and bereft when those
others departed. Society offers few obvious alternatives for
middle-aged women who find themselves in such positions and
may be starting to feel, 'Now I find that I — I want something
for myself too. I'm a human being and I'm thinking about
myself'. Bart comments of one woman, 'She agreed that a
paying job would boost her self-esteem. But what jobs are
available for a 40-year-old woman with no special training, who
has not worked for over twenty years?' Lacking real power and

control over their lives, sometimes manipulation and guilt were their only remaining weapons.

We saw in the first chapter how the hospital characteristically responds by an unquestioning reinforcement of the traditional values that led to the problem in the first place. Thus, these women are routinely assigned to programmes of cooking, shopping, and sewing, and their progress is measured by how well they do in these activities. Drugs and ECT are fairly standard. Psychiatrists, particularly male ones, often find these women as bemusing and frustrating as the husbands who suddenly find themselves with a weepy, despairing woman on their hands, and the tone of their letters often betrays this. Thus, one of Elaine's psychiatrists wrote to her GP, 'I spoke to her husband who seemed a fairly reasonable person, he had put up with Mrs Jones's relapses with relatively good humour and only occasionally criticized her for the difficulties she produced for the family', while in the opinion of another, 'She has many vague fears about the future . . . she really is too imaginative'. Exasperation and lack of comprehension on the part of the husbands is to some extent understandable; what is less excusable is the failure of the professionals to bring any greater degree of understanding to the situation. Apart from this, such women tend to be pushed to one side in the hospital as they are in life. They are viewed as cured if they manage to force themselves to take up their old roles as wives and home-makers, at whatever cost to themselves. Not believing that they deserve any better treatment, they pass through the psychiatric system without protesting or attracting the kind of attention that has been paid to less common but more dramatic conditions like schizophrenia.

None of this is meant to imply that it is a mistake for women to follow the traditional path of marriage and motherhood. Where this can lead to problems, though, is first, if it is a forced choice because it is the unquestioned thing to do and other options are not easily available; second, if these roles are carried out at the expense of the woman getting what she needs for herself, so that she is giving out of her own neediness and always putting herself last; and third, if the role of wife and mother is idealized by society while at the same time wives and mothers are devalued, unsupported, and blamed in reality. This is a dilemma currently faced by many women in their thirties, forties, and fifties, who on the one hand have followed the example set by their own mothers, while on the other they are presented with the tantalizing possibility of a different way of life, demonstrated by women they meet or read about or see on television and also by their own daughters. The two-way pull can be very powerful and painful.

Susie Orbach and Luise Eichenbaum, cofounders of the Women's Therapy Centre in London, have taken such observations several stages further to show how *all* women, whether psychiatric patients or not, share, at a very fundamental level, the struggle to come to terms with the conflicts and dilemmas of the woman's role. The 'depressed housewife' syndrome is just one manifestation of the confusions in which all women are caught up. As they explain, it is not a simplistic case of helpless women being victimized by wicked men. The dilemma is far more subtle and complex, and in fact it is mainly through the mother-daughter relationship that the female script is handed down from one generation to the next. The following exposition is paraphrased from their excellent book, *Outside In, Inside Out*.[3]

The central feature of the traditional woman's role is that she must be a wife, mother, and homemaker, and must take care of others emotionally. All these roles involve deferring to others, putting them and their needs first, 'not being the main actor in her own life'. She must live through others and shape her life through her partner (who must be male). There are various consequences to this. Because women are not seen as important individuals in their own right, because their work is repetitive and undervalued ('just a housewife', or a carer for elderly relatives, or else a secretary, domestic, shop assistant, nurse, all of which involve serving other people), they come to feel that they are insignificant, unworthy, and undeserving. Again and again, women put themselves down, hesitate to speak up for themselves, run down their achievements. Moreover they come to believe that their inadequacy is unique to them, that everyone else is managing far better, and in their isolation they take this as further proof of their worthlessness.

In order to take care of others emotionally, a woman has to develop exquisitely sensitive emotional antennae. Empathizing with others, picking up their feelings, intuiting reactions, and sensing emotional atmospheres all become second nature for most women. They can tell at a glance what mood their husband, child, or boss is in, and they become experts at guessing what is needed and supplying it. Here again, though, a woman must put herself last and not expect the same care for herself, and is left with a deep feeling of being unappreciated and uncared for.

These lessons in how to be a woman have to be learned mainly from another woman, mother, who has herself learned them as the daughter to her own mother. Here, a number of contradictory impulses come into play. If mother gives birth to a boy, he is clearly different, other than, separate from mother by virtue of his sex. If the child is a girl, though, mother will identify much more closely with her. Inevitably the feelings that mother has about herself at a very deep level will be *projected onto* the baby girl. In other words, because mother identifies so closely with her baby daughter, she will tend to see the baby more as an extension of herself than as a separate being. She will see parts of herself in her daughter, and some of her deep feelings about herself — her neediness, her wish to be cared for, her insecurity — will, without her being aware of it, be superimposed upon her baby. This leads to a very complicated situation. Mother wants to fulfil her daughter's needs and give her satisfaction and contentment, but it is very difficult for her to do this when her own needs have not been fulfilled. The sight of her daughter's neediness and vulnerability reminds mother of the needy, vulnerable parts of herself, which she has had to shut off in order to carry on her role of caring for others. This results in a sort of push-pull inconsistency in the mother-daughter relationship. When mother can see her daughter as a separate person, she can be responsive and loving and give her daughter the sense of security and well-being that she needs. At other times, it is as though the boundary between them dissolves and mother experiences her daughter and herself as having the same feelings, thoughts, and desires, almost as if she were an extension of the same person. When this happens, mother finds herself relating to her daughter in the same way as she relates to the locked-away, needy, little-girl part of herself which she has never come to terms with, and she ends up withdrawing from her daughter at one moment and becoming over-involved the next.

The effect on the daughter is very confusing — as it was when mother played out the same drama as a daughter to her own mother. What she learns is that it is all right to be needy, but not too needy; that she can strive for a fuller and more satisfying life than her mother, but that it is dangerous to go too far towards independence; that she can get emotional care and attention, but never quite as much as she needs; that she must seek happiness with a man, but must ultimately expect to be disappointed; that she must leave her mother to start her own family, but that all the same she should never quite separate from her. 'A son is a son till he takes a wife, but a daughter's a daughter all her life.' As daughter receives these crucial lessons in how to be a woman and how to set limits to her hopes and desires, she suppresses the parts of her that she has learned are unacceptable: the emotional cravings, and the anger and disappointments that come from never quite getting what she wants and needs in her first and most important relationship.

She comes to feel that there must be something wrong with who she really is, which in turn means there is something wrong with what she needs and what she wants. A process of feeling inauthentic develops. She feels unsure in her reactions and distanced from her wants. This soon translates into feeling unworthy and hesitant about pursuing her impulses. Slowly she develops an acceptable self, one which appears self-sufficient and capable; one that is likely to receive more consistent acceptance . . . she comes to feel like a fraud, for an external part of her is developing which is different from who she feels she is inside.[4]

Since the daughter never feels secure in herself at a deep level, she lacks the confidence to make a full separation from her mother. The world outside seems tantalizing but frightening, rather than a place that is full of exciting possibilities. Inside herself the daughter may never quite feel that she knows where she begins and mother ends; she may sometimes feel as if she is carrying mother around inside her. Both mother and daughter may need to stay close to each other so that neither loses their fragile sense of who they are, and this may make it very hard for daughter to join together with her husband if she marries. And if she has a daughter of her own, the whole cycle continues.

With all this in mind, we are in a better position to appreciate the intense separation difficulties of Jenny and her mother, Mrs Clark. A criticism that has been made of some of the family interaction views of schizophrenia — the writings of R. D. Laing especially — is that they do not describe anything that is particular to families where someone breaks down in a schizophrenic way; indeed, Laing's books are so compelling partly because we can all identify aspects of our own situations in them. Similarly, High EE (high emotional expression) has been found to be relevant to successful weight loss and recovery from depression as well as to schizophrenia. Indeed, I believe that the plight of mothers of children who are diagnosed schizophrenic is only one variation on a universal theme, although it is played out with a special intensity with these women, and certainly involves other factors such as unusual sensitivity on the part of the child. But it does not follow that family interactions play no part in the development of the problem. To take an analogy, out of a group of women living on an isolated housing estate, some may become depressed, some agoraphobic, some dependent on tranquillizers, while some will manage to make the best of the situation and settle in reasonably happily, and no doubt these differences could be related to all sorts of factors including, ultimately, their genetic and biochemical make-up. However it would be strange to argue that because the housing estate produced different reactions in different people, it could not be playing an important part in contributing to the problems; it would be even more strange to devote thousands of pounds to researching into the biochemistry of these women instead of examining the more immediate circumstances of their lives.

What we know about Mrs Clark, then, suggests that her way of relating to her daughter was a consequence of finding herself in the same trap described by Orbach and Eichenbaum and experienced by the women in Bart's article. She had followed the traditional path to marriage and motherhood under the influence of social and cultural expectations and a romantic dream. She transferred a dependency on her family to a dependency on her husband without any intermediate exploration of herself as an individual. When the dream turned sour, she found herself trapped in a failed marriage by her strong conviction that divorce was wrong, isolated in her neighbourhood, and with no interests outside the home. She invested everything in her children, and particularly in Jenny, who was most like her and the last child still at home. For Mrs Clark, Jenny's threatened separation faced her with unbearable isolation and emptiness. At a psychological level, Mrs Clark and Jenny were so tied up in each other's identity that separation threatened their very survival. In some cases, this turns out to be literally true. As we saw, medical model psychiatric treatment does not promote separation; instead, it legitimizes the sick role so that proper separation need never occur. But Scott found that if family work was carried out enabling the child to separate, the effect on the involved parent, usually the mother, could be devastating, confirming the two-way nature of the bond. Although many parents were eventually able to let their child go and find new fulfilment in their own lives, some mothers developed crippling mental or physical problems themselves after their child's departure.

There is a further consequence to the traditional family set-up where it is the mother's role to do most of the child-rearing, and that is that she tends to blame herself, and to be blamed by others, for any problems that the children have. This is very unfair, and prevents any analysis of why mothers are placed in such an impossible situation in the first place. It also ignores the role of the father, who plays an equally important part, if only by his absence or distance. The position of Mr Clark and of fathers in general will be discussed in the next chapter.

With individual variations, the same themes can be traced in all women. Here, for example, is the story of Sandra, a 22-year-old secretary, whose main complaint was not obviously related to women's role problems; she was haunted by the fear that she might become uncontrollably violent, perhaps towards her husband, but particularly towards babies and young children.

Sandra's story

Sandra said she had always been a shy, anxious sort of person. She lived at home with her parents and two sisters until she married her first boyfriend when she was eighteen. She idolized her husband, Rick; he was everything she wasn't — competent, easy-going, sure of himself. When Sandra came along to get help, she was feeling desperate. She was convinced that her thoughts about violence meant that she was going crazy. She might commit some terrible crime and be locked up in a mental hospital or prison. She was also terrified that Rick or her parents would die, or that she herself would die young and this would confirm her fear that she was doomed never to get what she wanted out of life. She wanted so much to be the perfect wife for Rick, but she was afraid he might leave her for someone more deserving.

Sandra had not been particularly happy at home, yet in some ways she and her mother were very involved with each other. For the first year of her marriage, Sandra missed her mother and family so much that she cried daily to go back to them. Her day-to-day life was a constant struggle to please people, a task in which she always felt she failed, despite the fact that she ended up doing twice as much as anyone else at work. In the supermarket she based her purchases on what she thought a really good wife would cook for her husband's supper. Sandra was convinced that everyone around her was coping far better. Ashamed of what she saw as her failings, she kept her worries and doubts to herself.

Both Sandra's and Rick's families lived nearby, and most of their social life revolved around them. It was a continual source of friction that Sandra wanted to visit her family every weekend. If she did not, she felt lonely and guilty, and this triggered her worries that they might die. But if she did go, it never turned out quite as she had hoped. Sandra's mother had given up a job she enjoyed when she married, in order to have children. Sandra's mother had been very close to her own mother and had suffered some sort of breakdown when she (Sandra's grandmother) died. On her visits, Sandra often wanted to confide in her mother, but somehow she rarely got the response she had hoped for. At other times she was aware of a vague feeling of wanting attention and not getting it, or she felt both guilty and irritated when her mother made remarks like: 'Never have children, they just grow up and abandon you.'

Sandra was coming along to therapy sessions once a week, sometimes with Rick when there were particular issues to sort out between them, but usually on her own.

As Sandra's therapy continued, a different side to her slowly emerged. Behind the part that was continually doubting, worrying, and striving to please, there was another part of her that sometimes dared to feel irritated, even angry, with the people round her. Rick was still almost perfect, but they had fallen into a pattern where he took the father role to her anxious child, and this sometimes went a bit too far. She didn't always like it when he made decisions on her behalf, or took over the driving with a patient sigh. One day they had their most serious row so far when for once Sandra stood her ground over something. It was a traumatic experience for her. She was petrified that Rick would leave her and she would go crazy left on her own, but they survived. At work Sandra said 'No' to a request for the first time, though not without difficulty. Most importantly, it became clear how desperately torn Sandra felt over the issue of whether or not to start a family. Her mother, despite her remarks about children who abandoned their parents, continually dropped hints about it, and even said openly that it was selfish of Sandra to be living just for herself. Sandra knew Rick wanted children and his mother was longing for a grandchild too. All her contemporaries seemed to be having babies, and the pressure to do the same was overwhelming. At the same time, Sandra found herself resisting the idea. It was hard for her to trust her own intuitions, especially when everyone around her was saying something different, but in the therapy sessions she dared to voice some feelings which at first seemed shameful and wrong to her. She didn't like the idea of all the responsibility of having a baby. She had a picture of everyone paying attention to the baby and not to her, and she thought she would resent that. She couldn't stand the idea of washing nappies. Sometimes she thought women only had babies because it was the thing to do. But she wanted to please Rick and her parents so much, and she felt so guilty for not doing so. She couldn't bring herself to tell Rick how she really felt, and somehow let him assume that they'd think about a family next year, and then she felt even more guilty. Was she wrong not to want a baby? Suppose she never wanted one? Such thoughts occupied a good deal of her time. The origins of her violent thoughts about babies and children became clearer. The sight of them triggered off the whole dilemma again, and with it a desire to kick the problem — and the babies — violently out of the way. By this time, though, Sandra was more likely to say 'Yesterday I felt like throwing a plate at Rick/Mum/my boss' than to report that for no apparent reason she had felt a terrifying impulse to pick up a sharp knife, an example of anger split off from its real source. She began to learn to recognize these frightening thoughts as a sign that she was feeling angry underneath and needed to express it. At the same time, she was realizing how much she disliked being a secretary. She simply didn't want to spend her day at other people's beck and call. She wondered whether she could give it up and spend some time working out what job she really did want to do. But her mother seemed to think this would be very selfish, and Rick might be angry because there would be less money coming into the house, and perhaps she should solve the whole problem by having a baby. On the other hand, she sometimes felt she had missed out by marrying so young. Part of her wanted to get out more, meet more people, try out new experiences.

Rick had quite a lot of difficulty adapting to the more assertive Sandra who was so different from the clinging, dependent girl he married, and Sandra had equal difficulty holding onto her own feelings, wishes, and beliefs in the face of the real or imagined disapproval of others. With many ups and downs, they struggled towards a more equal relationship, while Sandra was more able to stand back and separate from her family. As she grew in self-confidence and autonomy, her fears, guilt, and doubts correspondingly faded.

We can see how Sandra's story is a variation on the themes outlined by Orbach and Eichenbaum. Sandra's mother had never properly separated from her own mother (Sandra's grandmother) and in fact had a breakdown when she died. Sandra's mother had therefore been unable to give to Sandra the healthy sense of security that she needed in order to be able to separate and establish her own identity in her turn. If you have had enough of your emotional needs met in your family, you can leave easily; but the paradox is that if you are left empty and wanting, you will still be tied to the one place that is unable to give you what you need. Thus Sandra was continually drawn back home, hoping for some indefinable response that never came, and was continually disappointed. Because her mother had not been able to accept and love Sandra as she really was (since *she* had not been wholly accepted and loved by *her* mother and so on back up the chain), Sandra was left with a deep feeling that she was undeserving, not good enough, failing in some way. Moreover she was convinced that only she suffered these doubts and anxieties, but she missed the chance to confide in others and find out if this was really so because her shame forced her to put on a bright façade and pretend that everything was fine. In this way, women isolate themselves from each other. She tried to earn love by pleasing people and giving to them, first her family and then her husband, and developed an acutely sensitive awareness of how other people were reacting. But this did not in the end give her any deeper sense of security; she became even more split off from what she really felt and wanted, and because she never dared expose this side of herself to others, for fear of being rejected, it began to seem as though her real self must be crazy, violent, mad. If it ever slipped out, it would need to be locked away in a prison or mental hospital, as indeed it was already locked away inside herself.

If your sense of security is very fragile, the last thing you can risk is being angry with the people on whom you are so desperately dependent, because you cannot risk being abandoned by them. Sandra's sense of security when she was apart from her husband and family was so fragile that she constantly feared they would die. The most difficult feeling for her to express to them was anger, and so it had to be buried, to reappear in violent thoughts that seemed to have nothing to do with her. In the end it was this same anger, which she gradually learned to listen to and use constructively, that enabled her to achieve a degree of separation and autonomy.

In the long and difficult transition period, Sandra became very dependent on her therapist, and spent a lot of time trying to say what she thought the therapist wanted to hear and concealing the things she thought might shock or anger the therapist. Like most women who are deeply convinced of their unworthiness, she constantly feared that she was taking up too much time, that the therapist must be bored or have better things to do. It was very important for the therapist to offer uncritical acceptance and understanding of Sandra's hidden real self as it gradually emerged, and to encourage her moves towards independence. This was something Sandra's mother, despite her bitter regrets about giving up her job so soon to start a family only to be 'abandoned' by them, was unable to do. Intuitively, Sandra felt she needed to pursue her own interests and desires and to have some fun for herself before thinking about a family, and of course this is the best way of ensuring that you can give wholeheartedly to your children in the long run. But Sandra's mother put a great deal of pressure on Sandra to give up her 'selfish' job aspirations and have a baby at once. It was not surprising that Sandra felt herself doomed never to get what she wanted out of life, never able to step over the invisible barrier that prevents women from striking away from the traditional path. To be able to encourage this, Sandra's mother would have needed to face squarely up to the limitations of her own life, rather than persuade Sandra to validate the same way of life by taking it up too. If Sandra had given in, then the whole pattern would have been passed down to the next generation.

The pressures on Sandra to conform came not just from her family, but also from the whole culture. The number of women for whom choices are more open — going to college or university, sharing a flat with friends, living with a partner, moving many miles away from the family of origin — is still relatively small. For many there is still a powerful, often unquestioned assumption that young women will live at home until they marry in their early twenties, will set up home nearby, and fairly soon give up work to start a family of their own. This means that a lot of experimenting and growing up either simply does not happen, sometimes with disastrous results later on, or has to happen within the marriage, which is sometimes not strong enough to stand it. Sandra's and Rick's marriage was able to accommodate some changes, but having followed the cultural script so far, Sandra faced a head-on conflict when she wanted to wait a few years and pursue her career before taking the next step, and the strongest pressure to conform came from people around her who had conformed themselves and were in fact regretting it — her mother, and various women friends. It is very hard to react with unmixed pleasure when you see someone else heading down the path you half wish you had taken; it is far easier to drown your own doubts in an attempt to persuade them to join you on your path.

The traditional patterns are more common in the working classes, but it is not much easier for women at the other end of the sociocultural scale. In the last few years there has been a huge increase in eating disorders which appear mainly in women. Anorexia nervosa and bulimia nervosa are most commonly found in the middle and upper socioeconomic classes. It is women in these classes and this generation who are suffering most severely from the conflict between following the traditional expectations for women, as exemplified by their mothers, and the more recent but equally daunting image of the independent, successful, confident superwoman, complete with lovers and high-powered career. They are caught between two stools, unable to work out a middle path for themselves when faced with contradictory sets of messages. As a broad generalization, anorectics tend to react to this dilemma by trying to opt out of it altogether, starving themselves until they return to a childlike physique with no breasts, hips, or menstrual periods. Bulimics tend to be women who have apparently achieved many of the ambitions of the 'new woman' — they are often unusually intelligent, attractive, and successful — but inside, hidden from the world, they are caught between the old and the new roles, and express their anguish and confusion in alternate bingeing and vomiting.

Here is the story of Angela, a 19-year-old student who lost weight very rapidly during her first year at university.

Angela's story

Like Sandra (and indeed like all women at some level), Angela was closely emotionally involved with her mother, a house-wife who suffered from anxiety and depression. Angela's up-bringing was quiet and sheltered, and she, like her parents, was a practising Roman Catholic. The last words of Angela's grandmother (her mother's mother) to Angela were, 'Be good and look after your mother'. This hardly needed saying, since Angela was already devoting her life to these two aims. Angela and her mother could each tell what the other was feeling at a glance, and a circle of anxiety quickly developed where each was panicking about and trying to reassure the other. Angela's main desire was to please others, and again like Sandra this resulted in her losing sight of what she herself wanted, but despite constant striving she felt herself to be unworthy and wicked. This was reinforced by an interpreta-tion of Christian ideas which led her to believe that it was sinful to upset your parents, to be angry, or to cause anyone else to get angry.

When Angela went to university, she was faced with a whole new set of demands and expectations. She seemed to be surrounded by confident, outgoing girls who wore make-up, went to discos, and had boyfriends, all things which were alien and alarming to her. At the same time she felt that these were things she ought to do, indeed had to do, if she was to fit in and be liked. If everyone else was expecting this of her, they must be right. Unable to say no for fear of upsetting people, Angela found herself committed to half a dozen different societies and activities. Somewhere along the line she had picked up the idea that very soon she had to be independent, which was the last thing she felt inside. She interpreted being independent in a black-and-white fashion as competing successfully in this hectic world, making all her decisions entirely on her own, and never leaning on her parents again because to bother them would be wrong, and they might be upset or angry. There was also the idea that at some point she had to have a husband and children, although she could not imagine any man wanting her and felt she did not deserve a husband anyway.

Pushed and pulled by contradictory messages from others, unable to trust her own feelings or to say no to any of the demands placed on her, Angela felt her life was getting increasingly out of control. One of the few areas of her life over which she could exert some control was her eating. By rigorously limiting her food intake and starting a punishing exercise programme she gained a temporary feeling of achievement and power. The battle to subdue her body and her physical appetite also reflected her profound belief, reinforced by her religious ideas, that her real self was unworthy, selfish, and full of dangerous desires that had to be beaten down. The only time that she could allow herself to eat without feeling greedy was when her nails turned blue and pains ran up and down her legs.

When Angela came for therapy during her vacation, she weighed around 5 stone. Part of her treatment contract was an agreement that she would try to put on a pound a week in weight. The discussions, which sometimes included Angela's parents as well, centred around the meaning of Angela's self-starvation. On the one hand, her extreme thinness seemed to be one way in which she could demonstrate what she felt she should not be expressing openly: that she still wanted care, protection, and attention from her parents and felt very much like a little girl inside. It was a way of retreating from the whole world which seemed so frightening to her. On the other hand, starving herself was one of the few ways in which she could protest and rebel against everything that she felt was being forced upon her. In a way, it was her own bid for autonomy.

The same conflicts were evident in Angela's struggle to put on weight again. At first, she only felt safe if her parents determined exactly how much she needed to eat to put on a pound that week. She had no confidence in her ability to determine her own food intake, or her life. If she did dare to estimate for herself how much she should eat, she was terrified of getting it wrong and suddenly putting on 10 pounds, since her sense of control was as precarious in her eating habits as in her life. Progress was made when Angela was able to assert herself a little more with parents and friends, paralleled by her ability to decide what to eat even if it did not coincide exactly with her parents' wishes. She gradually came to appreciate that independence did not have to be the terrifying position of total competence and responsibility that she had visualized. She could move slowly towards it and move back again as she needed, rather as she was slowly putting on weight but retaining the right to stay the same weight for a week, or even drop a little, to reassure herself that she was still in control. Therapy took many months, during which Angela pursued a slow and sometimes erratic path towards greater self-confidence and autonomy.

Again, the issues that all women, psychiatric patients or not, have to struggle with, can be seen in Angela's story; separation from mother, achieving autonomy, compulsive caring for others, rejecting one's own feelings and needs, problems with asserting oneself and expressing anger. Angela's story also illustrates women's difficulties with having good things for themselves. Angela could only allow herself to eat if other people gave her food, or were eating as much as her; it seemed too greedy to reach out and take food for herself. Paradoxically, although most women are suffering from some variation of not getting enough for themselves emotionally, they often feel that they are already too greedy and selfish. They apologize to therapists for taking up too much time when there must be more deserving people to be seen; they take on other people's problems but do not ask for support in return because 'so-and-so has got enough on her plate already'.

Social pressures play a crucial part in anorexia too. Angela (like Jenny Clark) was acutely aware of the expectations placed on young women to look right, behave right, and compete for popularity, boyfriends, and careers. Her retreat from the world was paved by the current obsession with the shape and size of women's bodies. Perfect female bodies stare at us from every magazine and hoarding, while the measurements of Princess Diana's waist or the Duchess of York's hips are front-page news. In-depth discussions of the complex way women's bodies are treated in this society are available elsewhere.[5] Here it is enough to note the horrifying fact that in a recent survey of 348 schoolchildren between 12 and 18, psychologist Jane Wardle found that three-quarters of the girls (and over a third of the boys) tried to restrict what they ate in order to control their weight, and that these attitudes were often well established even in normal-weight girls of only twelve.[6] It is practically impossible to find an adult woman who feels at home and happy with her own, ordinary imperfect body. The fear, dislike, and sense of alienation that the anorectic feels for her body is only an extreme version of an attitude taught to all women. (Unfortunately, there are signs of a similar pattern emerging among young, career-minded men. 'Eating disorder clinics which never saw a male patient 5 years ago are now admitting a significant number of city professionals . . . The advertising pressure on men is mirroring what happened with women 10 or 15 years ago . . . Men with eating problems are driven to seek perfection . . . They can be very "with it" in the business world, but emotionally their lives are a mess.')[7]

How is anorexia treated in the psychiatric system? With the exception of a few specialist treatment centres, the approach is nearly always a behavioural one: that is, the symptom (loss of weight) is seen as the problem. Treatment is directed towards removing the symptom, i.e. persuading the patient to put on weight, and when she (or more rarely he) has done this she is regarded as cured and is discharged. Weight gain is produced by such methods as enforced bedrest while the anorectic patient is made to consume up to 3,000 calories a day, or by depriving her of all privileges (visits, books, telephone calls) until she earns them by reaching weight targets set by the staff. Some hospitals use powerful tranquillizing drugs to overcome the anorectic's resistance to rapid weight gain, or even give ECT. The very narrow definition of the problem allows psychiatrists to claim success for these methods; they certainly do make people put on weight. Their wider effects are less beneficial. Anorexia is all about control; to the anorectic, the rigid control she maintains over her weight is her only defence against chaos and despair. To have this defence seized from her as large amounts of food are virtually forced down her, with punishments ranging from isolation to ECT if she persists, is terrifying for her. Not surprisingly, many anorectics try to retain some control of the situation by any means left to them, such as secret vomiting or drinking large quantities of water before weighing sessions. This has earned them a reputation for being devious and manipulative patients, and Persecution may result. Since the underlying issues are not resolved, anorectics often lose weight again as soon as they are discharged, and may spend months or years being shuttled in and out of hospital to be fattened up and released again.

Treatments which focus solely on weight gain are falling into the same trap as the anorectic herself: they are treating her body as an object, as something separate from her as a person, to be forced into one shape or another without any regard to what this means for the young woman herself. Rather than helping the anorectic to accept and make friends with her body, the hospital may view it as a problem, an enemy, that has to be beaten down, the only difference being that the hospital wants it to be fat whereas the anorectic wants it to be thin. This in its turn is a reflection of the way society presents women's bodies as objects to be manipulated into the correct shapes to sell consumer goods, catch husbands, display the latest fashions, and so on. In addition the situation where powerful male doctors decide what is to be done to her body may echo and reinforce her fears about sexual relationships, that this is another area where she will feel used and not in control. The same attitudes underlie much of the academic research on anorexia, for which young women may be recruited to have electrodes attached to their hands, pulse and blood pressure taken, and haemoglobin and urea and cholesterol checked, in order to aid the classification of anorectics versus bulimics, dieters versus vomiters, without any regard to the person to whom the body is attached.[8]

There are sometimes emergencies where force-feeding is necessary to save an anorectic's life. These situations apart, a proper treatment contract which enables the anorectic to take an active part in her treatment and retain some control by negotiating how much weight she will be expected to put on and at what rate, is essential, although often lacking. In this way, weight gain or loss becomes a useful indication of how she is feeling, as Sandra's therapy showed, rather than the inevitable result of an externally imposed feeding programme. It can give a lead into the most important part of treatment: the search to uncover the meaning of the compulsive self-starvation. If this is done, the outlook is optimistic.

The rest of this book could be devoted to illustrating the

theme that women's role problems, as I have christened the mixture of psychological and social/economic pressures that women are subjected to, run like a thread through the stories of all female psychiatric patients and indeed of the lives of women in general to a greater or lesser degree. A young mother who was referred with panic attacks had been brought up on the dream of her own home and family, but the reality, isolated on a modern estate far from bus routes, with her husband out all day and no one to give her a break from her two toddlers, was an unpleasant shock. Another woman who became agoraphobic spent her life doing the chores for her husband and three grown-up sons. She said, 'I'm afraid that if I could get out of that front door, I'd never come back again'. Working with groups of overweight women, I discovered similar themes. Typically these were working-class women who had married young, devoted their lives to child-rearing, and now found themselves trapped in uncommunicative marriages, prevented by limited opportunities and lack of money and self-confidence from broadening their lives, and turning to food as a comfort and support. Another vast pool of female distress is concealed by tranquillizers such as Valium. Women are prescribed these drugs far more often than men (the ratio has been estimated at about two to one)[9] and this serves to obscure the underlying issues which are nearly always women's role problems. The 'That's Life' survey on tranquillizers found that most of the people who filled in their questionnaire were 'more readily identified by their normality rather than by their problems'. They described themselves as 'being happily married with two children, living in houses as owner-occupiers and enjoying an average standard of living'.[10] This strongly suggests that there is something very unsatisfying about the lives that normal, average women are expected to be content with. A famous study of working-class women in Camberwell, London, found that a quarter of them could be diagnosed as suffering from depression.[11] Factors such as being confined to the home looking after young children, and having no outside employment made them more vulnerable to depression. Women who take advantage of the sick role, like Jeanette, Fay, and Alice, whose stories were related in Chapter 3, are often trapped by women's role problems too. Sometimes they have devoted their lives to their families, only to find that there is no real niche in society for an unskilled, middle-aged, single woman if family life breaks down. Sometimes this realization makes them unable to face leaving an unhappy marriage. In either case, the sick role may be one of the few ways they can find care, attention, and a role for themselves. It can also provide indirect opportunities for venting the anger and frustration that women find so hard to express directly.

I have used some individual cases to illustrate the general theme that the psychiatric system reinforces the problems that women come along with by acting on the same assumptions that led to the problem in the first place. Certain psychological and social pressures lead to difficulties, and the hospital applies the same pressures, only more forcefully, to solve the difficulties. (Thus, a woman who breaks down partly as a result of being pressurized into the traditional role without getting enough care for herself may be forced into shopping and cooking programmes, with drugs to suppress her resistance, at the very time when she is most in need of care and understanding herself, and is labelled as a bad patient if she does not comply.) What most women in psychiatric hospitals need is first, to be helped to see that they are only part of the problem, and second, to get angry enough about it to make some real changes. The medical model cannot allow for this. Diagnoses are attached to individuals — there is no such thing as a medical diagnosis that includes a husband, children, parents, or wider society as an equal part of the problem. Thus the woman's belief that it is all her fault, which is preventing her from seeing possible changes and solutions, is reinforced. As for getting angry, this is the quickest way of getting yourself labelled as a bad and 'aggressive' patient and being Persecuted for it. Not complaining, obediently accepting the medication, orders, and opinions of others, is the behaviour that is approved and encouraged.

It has to be borne in mind that most psychiatric staff receive virtually no training in counselling or psychotherapy. Doctors and nurses do particularly badly in this respect. They are even less likely to get any specialist training in helping with such mainly female problems as anorexia, post-natal depression, being a victim of rape or of a violent spouse, or having an abortion or a miscarriage, let alone learning to look at psychiatric problems from the point of view of women's roles. It is only to be expected, therefore, that psychiatric staff will unwittingly reinforce the values of the society they come from, even where this actually makes the problem worse, since they have not attained any higher degree of critical awareness than their patients. The fact that this occurs is borne out by research studies. The classic one was carried out by Dr Broverman and her colleagues, in 1970,[12] and has since been confirmed by other studies.[13] Seventy-nine psychiatrists, psychologists, and social workers, both male and female, were given a questionnaire consisting of pairs of descriptions, for example, 'very emotional — not at all emotional' and 'not at all aggressive — very aggressive'. They were asked to tick the descriptions that represented healthy male and healthy female adult behaviour. They were also asked to tick the descriptions that fitted their idea of healthy adult behaviour (sex unspecified). The results showed that the professionals' ideas of what constituted a healthy mature male were very similar to their idea of a healthy adult. However, a healthy, mature woman, in their view, should be

more submissive, less independent, less adventurous, more easily influenced, less aggressive, less competitive, more excitable in minor crises, having their feelings more easily hurt, being more emotional, more conceited about their appearance, less objective, and disliking maths and science.

As the authors comment, 'This constellation seems a most unusual way of describing any mature, healthy individual'. This illustrates the trap awaiting women who come into contact with the psychiatric services. On the one hand, being independent, assertive, and adventurous is seen as abnormal for a woman, and discouraged in various ways. On the other hand, the more excitable, emotional, dependent behaviour that is expected of women is also seen as unhealthy, because the idea of emotional health for adults is virtually the same as the idea of the healthy adult male. Either way, the woman loses.

Other studies confirm the fact that women with less conventional lifestyles and attitudes fare as badly in psychiatry as their more conventional peers. Commenting on the fact that the less liberal counsellors in a group of mental health professionals saw a left-wing, politically active female as significantly more psychologically maladjusted than an identically described male client, researchers said that this result 'raises the spectre of covert discrimination against the "liberated" woman, unintentional though it may be, on the part of certain workers holding unsympathetic sociopolitical views'.[14] Other groups that are out

121

of step with approved social norms — gay women for example — may be subjected to similar covert discrimination, even if more explicit prejudice (seeing homosexuality as a mental illness which needs to be cured) has been abandoned, officially at least. These studies also remind us that the fact that a psychiatrist, psychologist, or whoever is a woman, gives no guarantee that she will be able to understand how a woman's emotional distress relates to the wider issues of women's roles: the female professionals had very similar views to the males, and female psychiatric staff are often just as guilty as the men of an unthinking reinforcement of traditional standards. When a woman presents with vague complaints of depression, irritability, tiredness, inability to cope, and protests tearfully, 'I've got a good husband and three children, I know I shouldn't be feeling like this', both male and female professionals are very much inclined to agree.

The more subtle messages of the psychiatric set-up are in line with all this. Women patients are unlikely to find many role-models of assertive, independent, and influential female staff during their stay in hospital. The most powerful, high-status, and well-paid individuals will be the predominantly male consultant psychiatrists, descending through the ranks to the lowest paid, low-status, predominantly female nurses, occupational therapists, secretaries, and domestics. In the health service as a whole, only 25 per cent of doctors are women although women make up 90 per cent of the nursing staff. Only 5 per cent of the higher paid senior administrative jobs are held by women.[15] In line with traditional labour divisions, it will be the female occupational therapists who supervise the cooking, knitting, and domestic activities, while the minority of male occupational therapists will probably be found in the woodwork or machine rooms.

Nurses are most exposed to the day-to-day stress of caring for patients, usually know them best, and yet have least say in their management. Very little provision is made for caring for the carers: support groups and places where they can talk about *their* distress are not seen as necessary to the job, while many of them find that their earnings will hardly stretch to outings, new clothes, holidays, or treats for themselves. In doing such a difficult job for so little recognition or reward, caring for others and yet not being adequately cared for themselves, they find themselves in the same dilemma as their female patients. Like these patients, they may accumulate frustration and anger at the exploitation and powerlessness of their position. However, they find it extraordinarily hard to use their anger constructively to assert their rights and opinions, individually or collectively, with the people further up the hierarchy, and in this too they resemble their female patients. Although there is usually much private grumbling among the nurses about the psychiatrists and their decisions, it is rare for them openly to challenge and disagree, however strongly they feel. It is a tribute to the nursing staff's dedication that so many of them manage to do such a good job despite the restrictions imposed upon them. The danger is that for a few of them, disillusionment and demoralization may take the form of venting their frustrations by Persecuting the bottom layer of the hierarchy, the patients.

A final case history illustrates what can happen when an ordinary, not very assertive woman enters a system with no treatment contract, psychotherapy, or whole-person, whole-system way of understanding people's problems.

Mary's story

Mary is a small, quietly spoken woman in her mid-thirties who was appallingly sexually abused as a child by her uncle. Many years later she found that she could not bear her husband to make love to her and felt violent if he even touched her. She did not make the connection between the two events and started to drink to deal with these frightening feelings. As she herself says, she is not the sort of person who questions authorities or experts, and so despite her reservations she came into psychiatric hospital when a psychiatrist recommended it.

'I was seeing Dr X for my drinking, and he suggested I become a voluntary patient. I refused — I didn't want to be classed as "mental". I never saw Dr X again until I was discharged six months later. I was admitted for two weeks' rest from the children and my husband. It was a nice break to be away from any sexual contact. I had no idea I was being put on pills, and then I was called suddenly to take them from the trolley. I wasn't told what they were for or what the side-effects were, nor was my husband told, and I felt unable to ask. I'm the sort of person that if a doctor tells me to take things I don't question it. Mind you, I would now — it's taught me a lot.

'I took another overdose because I was due for discharge. I didn't want to be here or at home, but being here was better than facing the problems at home. I was told to go to occupational therapy, but no one told me why I had to do it. I thought I was here for a rest. I know how to sew and do things like that already. I wasn't getting anything constructive to help me face my problems. I took another overdose so I was sent upstairs and my clothes were taken away from me because they said I was a danger to myself. They didn't figure out why I was taking overdoses, but I wasn't with anyone long enough to tell them. I would need to know someone before telling them about sex. You got to know a doctor for a few days and then they wouldn't be there. There must be a way of getting through to people that are shy and reserved, but if you sat back, you never saw anyone. I was here six months and I never went into the dining room. I was scared to walk in on my own. My husband brought meals in for me and no one ever noticed.

'My husband saw Dr X because I kept escaping. Dr X said I was the sort of person who had to disobey, but I'm not. My husband tried to explain, I'm the sort that obeys authorities. Apparently I was aggressive and unco-operative, Dr X told my husband; I wanted attention, but I'm the type who always sits at the back. A younger girl pushed her pills away and the nurses threatened to send her to St X's Hospital if she didn't take them. You can't get help with pills because you're all numb, you're still bottling things up. Really you need to get mad and shout your problems out. But you didn't — the nurses aren't battleaxes, but it was the whole attitude — you just did as you were told or you'll end up on a locked ward at St X's. Two nurses had a go at me one night when I'd taken an overdose — one grabbed my picture of my three children and shoved it in my face, and said, "Look what you've got — you keep on like this, my girl, and you'll go where you deserve". You're either ignored or treated like a child. The nurses check if you've had a bath, tell you to go and make your bed, you have to wait up until it's freezing before you get an extra blanket — silly things.

'I had ECT — I was advised to have it because it might do me good. It wasn't helpful, I don't know if it can do you any harm. I've lost a lot of memories and I can't remember a lot of the last three years. I remember taking my jewellery off, a bare draughty room and a white gown, a doctor came up behind me and the next thing I remember was being shaken to get out of bed. It frightens me now to think I let it go that far. I felt obliged to do it because I felt they knew what was best for me, and I was given no alternatives.

'With Dr X, I felt as if my time was up as soon as I sat down. I saw Dr Y twice in six months. The first time, she got me talking and I felt a lot better. Then I didn't see her anymore until I was discharged. I was left in mid-air. No one told me you had to make an appointment to see the doctors, or the difference between a psychologist and a psychiatrist. No one asked me if I wanted to talk to someone on a regular basis. I *wanted* to be helped, or I wouldn't have agreed to come in in the first place. I was terrified when I first arrived. There was a coloured man who kept telling me to get into bed with him, and you can't lock your door, so I just panicked. There was a girl with hair like you see on mad people on the TV, she just flopped around and had to be spoonfed. I thought "I'll end up like that". Things like that should be dealt with privately, for her sake as well as others. Some of the patients were in a dream, they'd sit next to you and mumble things you couldn't understand. You felt you were abnormal and this was the place for abnormal people, and yet they're *not* abnormal people when you get to know them, just normal people with a problem that perhaps just needs listening to. But you've got to find out what the problem is first — that's the hard part. The whole system is that you've got to conform, but when you think about it, the ones in here are non-conformists. Half of them don't need to come in in the first place. The general impression was that you go out and you come back in again, you're never completely free of the place. When I come back up to see John [the counsellor whom she was eventually referred to and who helped her to make sense of her horror of physical contact] I recognize all the old faces back in here again. I was called before a panel of it seemed like hundreds of people sitting in a ring and told I was going to be discharged and see John instead, but otherwise I think I might be still in here.

'I lost six months of my life in there. When I came out, I weighed 13 stone because of the tablets. It took me three years to come off the tablets, visiting my GP every month. I had withdrawal symptoms — palpitations, sweats. I had panic attacks and agoraphobia which I didn't come in with. I was scared to go out because everyone knew I'd been in the psychiatric hospital. I moved house to get away from the stigma, and I never hear from my old friends and schoolfriends any more. It was partly me cutting them off and partly them doing it to me. I got a new job but the story got out, and I feel I've been labelled.

'It makes me so mad and sad thinking back on it all. There was no need for me to come in in the first place. I just wanted someone with a bit of time, I needed someone to visit me at home perhaps, give me some moral support or arrange some help at home. I don't think I had a drink problem, because I know now *why* I was drinking. It's the doctors that want looking at — they can convince you that you're not well, that you need treatment, and then they don't give you any! People have the wrong idea about psychiatrists. It's not a nice man listening to you lying on a couch. They'd be much better off going to a person's home for half an hour, that's where they have all their problems. You can't judge people when they come to an office specially to see you.

'To get *worse* when you go into the place — there's got to be something wrong somewhere, hasn't there?'

6

Men's role problems and psychiatry

A recent television programme[1] brought together a group of men to discuss their lives as males. When they were asked what was expected of them as men, they came up with the following list:

To provide for the family.
Never to cry.
To be reasonable and rational.
Never to show fear, no matter how afraid I am.
To have a career.
To be competitive.
Not to show any weakness.
Not to be feminine.
To be the one that doesn't crack under the strain.
To settle down.
To be the father and apply discipline.
To marry and preferably have a son.
To be a lad.
To know about mechanics.
To be a painter, decorator, plumber, handyman, and fix the car.

If women's lives are powerfully and often destructively shaped by the expectations of what is appropriate for their sex, then the same is equally true for men. The resulting division of skills, obligations, and attributes between the sexes means that both men and women are handicapped in growing to their full potential. This can have devastating effects upon them, their relationships, their children, and the society in which they live.

There are always many individual exceptions to general rules, and in recent years the rules governing sex roles have been relaxed a little, especially among the middle classes. Paradoxically, one of the factors that prevents the rules actually being overthrown, rather than just weakened, is the belief that the change has now happened, that the sexes have achieved equality. This ignores the fact that in most sections of society all the old rules are still in force, that in the middle classes they are not absent but merely more subtle, and that men have hardly begun to question their roles at all. To summarize the situation briefly and in general terms:

Women are powerful in the family, men are powerful in the outside world

There is an old joke in which the wife says 'I make all the minor decisions like where we live and what schools the children go to. He makes all the important decisions about defence policy and the national debt.' It is still generally mother who is blamed if the cornflakes run out and the clothes aren't collected from the laundry, and who knows the small details of the children's worries, preferences, and friendships. Correspondingly it is the father who bears the ultimate responsibility for supporting the family financially. How both sexes lose out is that mother may end up trapped and frustrated in a restricted life of repetitive chores and demands, unable to use her talents in a wider sphere. A wife who works outside the home as well tends to add this job to her existing tasks, rather than shedding any. Meanwhile father may be increasingly ground down by an uncreative job, cut off from getting to know his own children as they grow up.

Men are allowed to be angry; women are allowed to be vulnerable

It is expected that men will assert themselves, make demands, show their anger. It is not shameful for a woman to confess doubts, fear, or loneliness, to cry, and to ask for help and comfort. How both sexes lose out is that men may find it impossible to admit to anything that seems like weakness, so that all their hurts are channelled into aggression or violence, whereas women may become overwhelmed by their self-doubts and fears and be unable to use their anger constructively to assert themselves and change their situations.

Women are permitted to be emotional, while men pride themselves on being rational

Women have a rich emotional life; they can be elated, tearful, loving, fearful, tender, excited. Men are expected to think, analyse, label, and solve problems by reason and intellectual understanding. How both sexes lose out is that women may be subtly discouraged from knowing facts about the world — science, politics, current affairs — so that their experience remains private, cut off from and ignored by the wider world; while much male-dominated expertise in these fields fails to take account of the human feelings of the people it affects.

Men have power, women have relationships

Men are far more likely to win positions of power in the wider world as politicians, consultants, lawyers, heads of companies, and so on, while in the home their power derives from physical strength and from being the main wage-earner. Women know how to make close and confiding relationships, especially with other women, where they can share the most intimate details of their lives. How both sexes lose out is that women are disenfranchised in the world in which they live, so that their priorities and values are ignored (as, for example, in the lack of child-care facilities which ties many women to the home), whereas men are often without a single male friend to whom they can really open their hearts in times of need.

Women are encouraged to care, men are expected to compete

Through caring for others, either their families or in their work in the 'caring professions', women get deep satisfaction. Men, much more than women, enjoy the feeling of achievement from making their mark in the wider world. How both sexes lose out is that women, as we have seen, are unable to compete for the care that they need for themselves; while for men, competition can become an end in itself, creating a ruthless working environment where lives and careers can be destroyed overnight for the sake of the business.

The irony is that in many ways both men and women end up in similar positions, although they approach those points along different paths. For example, both men and women are alienated from their bodies, although in different ways and for different reasons. Women expend large amounts of energy on disliking their bodies for not living up to whatever the current ideal is, and trying to force them into shape with diets, exercise, and uncomfortable clothes. But although men are spared most of these excesses, they are also discouraged in subtle ways from enjoying the sensual pleasures of soft clothes, perfumes and body lotions, hugs and strokes, and other forms of pampering that are permitted to women. For a man, even taking care of his body with rest, nourishing food, and good medical care can seem a rather suspect activity compared to a more manly striving and testing in the face of a bravely borne physical hardship. To take another example, women often feel that their sexuality and sex lives are not under their control. They are encouraged to present themselves as desirable and sexual, while at the same time there is a strong taboo against openly and straightforwardly approaching men they may be interested in. Their role is the frustrating and degrading one of waiting to be selected, hoping that their signals are obvious enough to be read by the man of their choice while not being so overt as to threaten him or scare him off. Having hooked him, the average woman continues to find it very hard to make a clear and direct request for what she wants, or a firm and definite refusal of what she does not want, sexually or otherwise. But men also lose control of their sexuality. For an adolescent boy, sex is often not so much an expression of love and a desire for closeness as a move in an intensely competitive game with his male peers. There is no easy way to opt out of the terrifying obligation to approach girls, risking humiliation and rejection in front of one's friends, and those who fail this test of manhood carry a lasting sense of inferiority. This means that men too lose sight of what they actually want out of sexual relationships, as opposed to what they think they *ought* to want and do in order to keep up with what they imagine everyone else is wanting and doing. A myth has grown up about men's powerful and uncontrollable sex drive, and indeed it may have a compulsive quality if a man is constantly trying to prove his manhood through it, and if it is one of the few ways in which men can satisfy their need for intimacy and physical closeness.

The list could be extended with numerous variations on the theme that men *do* while women *feel*. Each sex's strengths are equally valuable, although different. Each side is needed to complement and balance the other. However, since society's values are by and large the traditionally masculine ones, the feminine point of view is often seen not as complementary, but as inferior. Thus, men's talk about things and events (cars, sport, politics) is important, real talk while women's fascination with feelings and relationships is 'nattering', 'rabbiting', or 'gossip'. Men have jobs while women just do housework, which somehow does not count as a proper job at all. The female-dominated caring professions are grossly underpaid compared to the competitive, male-dominated world of business and finance.

Where women have an enormous advantage over men is that in being allowed to retain their emotional lives, they have also been able to *feel* frustration at the restrictions and obligations of their role, and as they have gained more economic power and independence they have been able to get on and *do* something about it as well. Men, on the other hand, tend to be not only constricted by their role but, as part of the role, cut off from their feelings about this constriction. They may be only fleetingly aware of the loneliness of having no friends to whom they can reveal their deepest fears and hopes, or of their anger at spending forty years in an exhausting and repetitive job in the name of family responsibility, or of the strain of presenting a tough, competent façade in order to compete with other men, or the burden of constantly defending their manhood against the dreaded accusations of 'sissy' or 'coward'.

While researching her excellent book, *Men* (and it is interesting that it is often *women* who have raised men's issues for discussion), Mary Ingham found:

> The really major problem of writing about men is that the majority of men do not think they have a problem. . . . I had met a selection of agreeable, fairly normal family men who had reached the age of 35, who cut the lawn, washed the car, played the occasional game of squash, liked to watch television and go out for a meal with friends, and were fairly

contented with where they had got in their work. . . .
Although a large number of men worked long hours, either
because they needed the overtime pay or because the responsibilities of their job demanded it, few showed any real resentment of this intrusion into their personal lives.[2]

Eventually she realized that 'I had what I now know to have
been a very naive crusading spirit which impelled me to find out
what made men tick, what was vulnerable about them. I
imagined it would just take a sympathetic female ear and they
would bare their souls, just like women do.' Gradually, though,
she began to

> look at all the material I had gathered in a very different light.
> What if men were feeling all the stresses and strains, but
> plastering them over, covering them up in a classic defensive
> way? I had expected men to explain their dilemma, to *tell* me
> what was wrong, to be consciously aware of it and able to
> articulate it, give it a name. . . . For men, the problem not
> only has no name but is not recognized as a problem.[3]

Men who are reading this chapter and exclaiming,'What a
load of rubbish!' may like to consider whether this reaction is
part of the phenomenon that Mary Ingham is describing.
All this makes it very hard for men to welcome the women's
movement. As far as some men are concerned, they stand to lose
the automatic provision of food, clean laundry, and so on, while
being expected to take on a whole lot of unwelcome new tasks,
like ironing and changing nappies, under the instruction of a
new breed of bossy women who may also start challenging them
at work. Sometimes they grumble that women have always been
the real bosses behind the scenes anyway, getting their own way
by feminine wiles. They fail to appreciate that this kind of
manipulation is often the only option left when more direct
power is denied to women. Men also find it hard to appreciate
the enormous benefits that the women's movement can bring
them; the freedom to discover and accept their own feminine (to
them 'weak') side, and to share or shed some of their burdens
and responsibilities.
In this respect it is unfortunate that there is an anti-men
flavour to some (though not all) feminist thinking. Many
women have good reason to be angry with men (and vice versa),

and yet this anger needs to take into account the fact that men, too, are constrained by powerful and crippling sex role expectations. The fundamental task for both the women's movement and the still comparatively recent men's movement is for each sex to recognize their own contribution to the destructive game and work out ways of changing it. Some men have recoiled from the whole idea of feminism before the furious accusations blowing towards them from the women's camp, while others have gone to the opposite extreme, and formed men's groups where they sit around castigating themselves for being so wicked to women and desperately working out ways to atone for it. Neither position is particularly constructive. A more recent trend in the men's movement is for men to trust women to have the courage and determination to work out their own way forward, while recognizing that the most helpful thing men can do, for women but equally importantly for themselves, is to meet together to work on the ways men are oppressed and to find positive ways of growing and changing.

Not nearly as much has been written on the psychology of how men learn the lessons of manhood as on the corresponding situation for women. (Indeed the content of this chapter, which has turned out to be almost as much concerned with women as with men, reflects this fact.) However, it is possible to put together some of the pieces of the jigsaw.

We saw in the previous chapter some of the consequences of the fact that women are the main caregivers to their children, that only women mother. Hence, 'mothering' has quite different implications from 'fathering'. This basic fact has been accepted unquestioningly for generations, and we are only just starting to look at its effects on human development.

For women, as we saw, one result is that they find it very hard to separate fully from their mothers, being so closely identified with them in this first, intense, one-to-one relationship where father is only an intermittently present background figure. On the other hand, since mother and daughter are the same sex, it is comparatively easy for little girls to learn the important lesson of what sex they are and what it means to be a girl — they get this experience directly from mother, even though this is at the expense of later difficulties in achieving independence. The situation is different for little boys. In order to learn what it means to be a boy, and enter the world of men, boys have to reject much of the close, intense attachment to and identification with mother that makes up the very earliest stage of life. Mother is a woman and sooner or later the little boy has to leave her apron strings and grow up like father and other men, who have up till then only played a distant part in his life. It has been suggested that this difficult and painful shift in his relationships and attitudes, taking place at a very young age, has lasting consequences for the little boy and later the man.[4] The slow but relentless initiation into the world of men can feel like a devastating rejection and abandonment by the first woman in his life, his mother. The blow is made doubly harsh by the fact that not only is he losing his first intense relationship, but also everything that goes with that feminine world — closeness, touch, feelings, intimacy — is being defined as out of bounds. He is cut off not only from his mother but also from his own feminine side, on pain of being taunted as a 'mummy's boy' or 'pouf'. Studies show that the lessons are learned early (gender identity is firmly established by 2½ years old), and are reinforced, even if unconsciously, in all areas of the little boy's (and the little girl's) life. For example, it has been demonstrated that mothers tend to leave boy babies crying while girls are picked up;[5] that when the same 6-month-old infant was presented to eleven mothers, their response to it was very different according to whether they were told it was a boy or a girl ('boys' were handed trains while 'girls' were given dolls and described as softer, more delicate etc.);[6] that nursery-school teachers encourage passivity, assertion, and aggressiveness quite differently according to whether these qualities are displayed by boys or girls;[7] and so on. In an experiment where twenty pairs of 9-year-old boys were left, in turn, to play in a room, they turned at once to the toys, displaying no personal curiosity, asking no personal questions, and conversing only about the technical problems of Lego-building. Twenty pairs of girls, on the other hand, used the Lego merely as something to pass the time while each got down to finding out where the other lived, what their school was like, what they disliked in their teachers, and all about each other.[8] A study of children seen at a child guidance clinic found that the majority of them had been referred when they deviated from the kind of behaviour expected for their sex.[9] There are numerous similar studies demonstrating that even though there *may* be innate psychological sex differences, the most important variable is the gender role that the child is assigned to. On building sites and in public schools the lessons are the same.

The end result, it has been suggested,[10] is that the little boy (and later the little boy inside the grown up man) is left with an unfulfilled longing for the intimacy he once had, together with a deep suspicion of the kind of closeness that might awaken his buried emotions and make him vulnerable to being rejected again. The whole dilemma is sealed over and probably lost to consciousness behind the pursuit of male activities, many of which seem designed to blot out uncomfortable feelings: alcoholism, workaholism, and so on. The conflict may be re-awakened later in his relationships with girlfriends or wife, when he may find himself cutting off emotionally, backing away from commitment or expressions of feeling, in a way that is as bewildering to him as to his partner. The tragedy for many men is that while at a deep level they long for intimacy, they are often hopelessly ill-equipped to achieve it, the whole world of emotions being an alien and frightening one to them. This difficulty is paralleled by women's problems in achieving autonomy, and both dilemmas can be traced back to the practice of having mother as the main or only caregiver while father is pushed to the edge of the family circle.

The world of men into which the little boy is initiated is in many ways a harsh one. A counsellor in the men's movement pointed out to me the enormous significance of the fact that men are brought up with the expectation that as adults they will be prepared to kill other men. The thought of women being trained to kill other women is quite horrific — and yet where men are concerned, we accept this fact and along with it a very high level of day-to-day violence (punch-ups, muggings, wife-beating, vandalism, and so on). So far, the best solution that society can come up with is calls for more violence in the form of short sharp shocks for offenders, stiffer prison sentences, capital punishment, and other punitive measures.

One of the penalties of belonging to the sex that tends to *do* rather than *feel* is that the blame for huge numbers of appalling deeds (wars, torture, rape, assault, and so on) is laid at your door. Thus, men tend to carry round a belief that they are basically *bad* as opposed to women's feeling that they are basically *worthless*. However, change cannot take place from a position of blame, guilt, and self-hatred. This does not mean that we should let people off the hook for destructive behaviour — men (and women) are not merely helpless victims of society any more than they are the evil creatures that a minority of

135

feminists would have us believe. There is a danger of the next switch in the Rescue game occurring, as women, who have traditionally taken the Victim role, turn to Persecute the men who have traditionally either Persecuted or Rescued them. What is needed, as was described in the chapter on treatment contracts, is a recognition that men (like women) are responsible for their behaviour, and at the same time in need of compassionate understanding of the processes that led up to that behaviour. When this is coupled with a belief that men (like women) are fundamentally good and loving and can be helped to get in contact with the good and loving parts of themselves again, then real change is possible. For men who are in trouble, this means letting go of a lot of deeply buried fear, grief, and anger, and rediscovering their feminine side.

Where men and women both run into problems is, as I suggested at the start of the chapter, when the traditionally masculine qualities that men are encouraged to develop are not balanced by the traditionally feminine ones (and vice versa for women). So, if men are permitted to be aggressive, but are discouraged from expressing fear, hurt, grief, tenderness, or neediness, all these may be channelled into rage or violence, or else take their toll in ulcers and coronaries, since there is no other outlet for them. We saw how women who are overwhelmed by women's role problems may end up in psychiatric hospitals where they get more of the treatment that led to the problems in the first place, i.e. a heavy reinforcement of the traditional role. Men are more likely to end up in the ultra-macho environment of the prison, where the toughness and brutality that led to *their* problems will be equally heavily reinforced. Women end up in psychiatric hospitals where they are punished for what they *feel*; men end up in prisons where they are punished for what they *do*.

What does all this mean for men and psychiatry? Of course there are also plenty of male patients in psychiatric hospitals, and their position will be discussed shortly. Very often, though, men are the hidden other halves of the problems that bring women along to the psychiatric services. This is to be expected if women are indeed more in touch with their feelings and more able to admit to having problems and ask for help.

The socialization of women which encourages the expression of emotions and discussion of personal feelings and problems, accounts for women more frequently labelling themselves, being labelled by others, and consequently appearing more frequently in mental health statistics.[11]

Frequently, though, the woman who is identified as the 'sick one' or the 'crazy one' is in fact carrying the problem for both partners or even for the whole family. Women are quick to blame themselves for everything, and men can preserve their image of being capable, rational, and strong by going along with this, consciously or unconsciously. While this enables male partners to avoid the painful business of admitting their own shortcomings, it also means that their difficulties, which may be as great or greater than those of the woman, are not resolved or even recognized.

The story of Elaine Jones described in Chapter 1 is a clear illustration of this. Elaine went through appalling suffering during her fifteen years of recurrent depression, but there were signs that her husband too, although not officially labelled as ill, had been through his own form of torment. We know that he had spent the greater part of his life shackled to an exhausting and poorly paid job to fulfil his male responsibilities as provider for the family. He had also had many years of stress over his wife's depression and had taken over care of the children during her frequent hospital admissions. The rest of his background is unknown; the professionals who treated his wife did not see it as relevant. Mr Jones was left to deal with his fear and despair in the traditional masculine way: silently, and on his own. This left him in an impossible situation. Not only was he ground down by the enormous burdens he had carried over the years, but he was also completely unequipped to adapt to his wife's greater assertiveness and her need for him to understand her feelings and communicate with her on an emotional level. He could not even admit to his own feelings, or take advantage of his wife's plea to confide in her when she sensed his despair, and he refused point-blank to attend a joint therapy session or do anything else that meant acknowledging his own vulnerability and need for help. Trapped in his male role, his only outlet was the common male one of venting his feelings in violent rages, while his body developed very severe ulcers. Mr Jones badly needed help in his own right, but the psychiatric staff were no better at recognizing his need for help and offering it than he was at asking for it.

137

Shadowy and poorly understood male figures have been glimpsed in the background of several of the stories from earlier chapters. Fay, who adopted the sick role and eventually became a long-stay patient, had a husband who seemed to have some investment in keeping her sick. What this investment might have been was never investigated or discovered. George, the husband of Alice, another 'sick role' patient, had numerous problems of his own, as was starting to emerge in marital therapy before medical model treatment was reintroduced and his part in the problem was screened out again. In the last chapter, I described how women who are seriously overweight are often suffering from women's role problems. In group sessions, the picture that emerged of their boyfriends, husbands, or ex-husbands was of men who were also trapped: too tired after a day's work to do anything but watch TV, or too dispirited by unemployment to take part in family life; sometimes locked in a grief they could not express for a dead relative, or suffering from sexual problems for which they refused to seek help. Their wives turned to food as a substitute for the missing intimacy and affection, while the men might turn to drink, or simply sleep the day away. For these men there was an extra layer to the trap; while their wives were able to find enormous relief and support in sharing their problems in a group or among friends, the men could not do the same, nor could they take advantage of their wives' repeated pleas to 'tell me what's the matter'. Frequently and frustratingly, male partners will refuse point-blank to come along for therapy with their wives or girlfriends. 'He doesn't believe in all that stuff — he thinks it's all a lot of rubbish. He says we ought to be able to sort out our problems on our own instead of asking a stranger', their wives and girlfriends will report, so that the psychiatric hospital may to some extent be forced to go along with the notion of the woman being the only one in need of help. However, dealing with one partner out of necessity is a very different matter from basing the whole treatment on the assumption that one person is the whole source of the problem. Thus, although Elaine's husband refused to come along for joint sessions, therapy was based on the belief that he and the rest of the family did play a crucial part in her difficulties. Women who initially describe their partners as 'easygoing, never worries about a thing', often change during therapy to saying, 'Honestly, I think he's got more problems than I have. He's the one who should be sitting here, not me'.

Equally sad is the situation of the father of Jenny Clark (the young woman who was diagnosed as schizophrenic). One result of having different roles for each sex is that heterosexual relationships contain a great deal of disappointment. We saw how women grow up with a deep sense of neediness and being misunderstood and uncared for. One of the ways they try to fill this very painful emptiness inside them is by a search for 'Mr Right', who will at last fulfil their needs, understand and cherish them, and give meaning to their lives. Popular culture — magazines, books, pop records, advertisements, films — reinforces this search at every turn. Eventually the young woman meets someone she is able to cast in the role of Prince Charming. The younger and less experienced she is, the more complete the illusion is likely to be, although unfortunately it is deeply rooted in older and more cynical women too. Of course, he cannot fulfil her unconscious hopes and needs. Probably no one could, since she is expecting something of him that in the end she has to find ways of doing for herself, but he is particularly ill-qualified for the task she has unwittingly set him, because he cannot deal with his own needs and feelings, let alone with hers as well. She finds that her women friends still understand and communicate with her better than her husband, while he is bewildered and angered by demands from her for something he finds hard to comprehend, let alone supply. She has in effect been asking him to Rescue her, and when this fails, she may turn to Persecuting him — ridiculing him, pushing him to the edge of the family circle, and seeking her fulfilment through her children instead. Jenny's mother married young from a very sheltered background, and this drama seems to have been played out in Jenny's family. Where it is the son rather than the daughter who is diagnosed as schizophrenic, a common pattern is that the son has been required to make up for his father's failure by acting as a kind of substitute partner for his mother, and has been unable to break away and join the adult male world along with his contemporaries. Very little was known about Mr Clark. His contribution was ignored by the hospital as it was in the family where, a pathetic figure, he hovered ineffectually in the background. Like many fathers, he was cut off from real closeness with his children, but his role was extremely important if only because of its absence, which contributed to the damaging lack of balance in the family relationships.

Then there are the more sinister male figures from Chapter 2 of Bill, who seemed to want his downtrodden wife Susan locked away so he could carry on having affairs, and the violent father of Andy, who left his son with such a burden of guilt and hatred, while in Chapter 5 we heard about the uncle who subjected Mary to horrific sexual abuse. Again, we have to remember that only people who have themselves been brutalized are capable of acting so brutally, though this does not absolve them of responsibility for their actions. A counsellor who works with violent men told me that in every case he had found two things to be true: first, that these men had been victims of violence themselves, even if this was done in the name of 'discipline', and second, that they passed on *less* violence than had been inflicted on them. Men who behave like this are full of the buried grief, loneliness, and fear which goes along with the harshest imposition of the male role.

The distribution of psychiatric problems between the sexes tends to reflect the different ways men and women are socialized. Thus, while women are more likely to become overwhelmed by their feelings and hence suffer higher rates of depression and neurosis, the so-called 'personality disorders', involving anti-social and irresponsible behaviour, and alcoholism, are much commoner in men.[12] But for whatever reasons men present themselves to the psychiatric services, the same male role themes tend to form part of the problem. John from Chapter 2, who was unable to grieve for his dead father and coped with his feelings by drinking, is a case in point. He and his brother had lived in the same house as they watched their father slowly dying, but when asked by his therapist if they had talked over their grief together, John made the classic reply, 'You can't talk to your brother about things like that!'

One situation that deals men a particularly severe psychological blow is unemployment. Studies have found significant increases in symptoms such as anxiety, depression, insomnia, irritability, lack of confidence, listlessness, inability to concentrate, and general nervousness in unemployed men, as well as alcoholism, raised blood pressure, and heavier smoking,[13] while 'the unemployment index is the strongest predictor of changes in the suicide rate, having a substantially greater impact on male suicide rates than on female suicide'.[14] Brenner's important work in 1973, since confirmed by other studies, found a link between economic recession and higher rates of admission to New York mental hospitals for which the most likely explanation is that economic stress and unemployment lead to an increase in psychiatric symptoms.[15]

There are obvious reasons why life on the dole should be depressing: less money and all that it entails, lack of goals and structure to one's life, and so on. However this is not a complete explanation. A small subgroup of the unemployed manage to keep active and enthusiastic and to create goals and opportunities for themselves. 'These unemployed people drew a clear distinction between work in general, to which they were strongly committed, and employment to which they were less committed.'[16] Nor does it explain why the association between psychological well-being and paid employment fails to hold for women as a group, although single women and principal wage-earners do show a similar pattern of effects.[17] At least part of the harmfulness of unemployment comes from the way it is perceived by the individual and the people around him, and this is where men, whose identity is so closely tied up with work, are hit so hard.

> Traditional men still define themselves in terms of their work: 'I 'am a builder . . . an engineer . . . a journalist . . . a salesman. . . .' . . . Boys are instructed from birth that you can only be somebody if you make external achievements which accredit you with power, financial or social. The corollary to this is that you cannot amount to anything in yourself, indeed you are not a *person* unless you have influence over some portion of the world at large.

Loss of this role is

> an existential and not just an economic problem. If such a man is hit by unemployment and cannot find a new role in life he is confronted with loss of both working faith and identity.[18]

This commitment to the idea of having a proper job remains, despite alarming statistics about some of the consequences of being *in* work. 'Executive burnout is one of the commonest causes of hypertension and infarction. It can be a killer.'[19] In Britain, an estimated 2,000 workers died from an injury sustained on the job, another 1,000 die from an industrial disease, and a million take sick leave because of an industrial illness, every year.[20] The so-called 'Type A' personality, highly competitive, compulsive about deadlines, and pushing himself relentlessly without regard to fatigue, has been found to be the most prone to heart attacks, and yet these characteristics are only a slightly more extreme version of the traditionally admired masculine approach to life.

Here are some further brief illustrations of men's problems as they are presented to psychiatry:

Jim, forty-two, was troubled by giddiness, fears of fainting, and acute anxiety in many situations, particularly at the market stall he ran on Saturdays and Sundays. From Monday to Friday he worked for the gas board, a poorly paid job that he detested. He could make far more money from his weekend stall, but he needed the security of a regular income in case the market trade dried up. So he worked seven days a week, and rarely had enough energy to go out socially or do anything except collapse in front of the television. His wife had recently had a minor breakdown after the death of her mother, on whom she had been very dependent. Apart from needing to learn some behavioural techniques for coping better with his anxiety, the most obvious way of understanding Jim's symptoms was that he was working himself far too hard, and that his symptoms were a form of protest. Yet Jim flatly refused to concede this. Most of his mates were doing the same to make ends meet, he argued, apparently unable to appreciate that having to do something for financial reasons does not necessarily mean that your body will happily go along with it like an obedient machine. He did not see his wife's unhappiness as having any particular effect on him, although of course he would rather she felt better, and nor did he believe that spending five days a week in a job he detested could produce symptoms of stress — everybody else at work felt the same, he said, and they all coped all right. (To an outsider, of course, Jim also looked like one of the copers, since he was much too ashamed to confide his difficulties to anyone.) Like many men who come for help, Jim simply wanted his distressing symptoms removed so that he could carry on the same lifestyle as before. He had never questioned his lifestyle, and could/would not see how it could have anything to do with his problems.

David was a young business executive whose driving ambition had won him a high-ranking position and an even higher salary by the age of 28. He got an enormous thrill from the challenge of winning new orders for his firm, and the long hours and the intense pressure to keep up were all part of this exciting lifestyle. The car, the salary, and the status were all evidence of his success, and this was very important to David, since he had always been intensely competitive. Indeed, competing was a theme in most areas of his life. His recreation was a hard game of squash, which he had to win, or swimming against the clock. His social life was a matter of making the right contacts and keeping up appearances. David wasn't aware of being unhappy with any of this, but his body was beginning to protest, and he developed very severe ulcers. He could not switch off from his work when he got home and could not get to sleep at night, haunted by the fear that he would not be able to keep up, his success would slip away, and he would be exposed as a fraud and a failure after all. He kept going until one day he was overcome by an inexplicable wave of depression and loneliness. Fearing that he was on the edge of a breakdown, he asked his GP to refer him for psychological help.

Alan, 35, worked in an insurance company. He had suffered from various digestive problems, for which his GP could find no physical cause, for several years. The striking thing about Alan, an intelligent and courteous man, was his inability to describe any feelings whatsoever. He simply was not aware of having any. This had never struck him as a problem until he was invited to join group therapy sessions, where he seemed bewildered and confused by what went on (though when he was asked to describe this experience, he quickly rationalized it away by explaining that he had complete trust in the therapist's professional judgement about the usefulness of the group). Alan could not understand the point of everyone sitting around going on about their feelings. He characteristically responded to any expression of emotion by immediately producing a practical solution, and kept asking the therapist if he had worked out the answer to his (Alan's) problems yet. Frustrated by his inability to relate on an emotional level, the group members started to pick up on Alan's body language as a clue to his buried feelings. Noticing that he was clenching his fist at one point, they asked if he was feeling angry. Looking down at his hand with some surprise, Alan admitted that perhaps he might have been feeling a shade irritated. Later he let slip a piece of personal information, that his wife was six months pregnant, and was taken aback when the group expressed its surprise that he hadn't thought to mention this important fact before. It was in small steps like this that Alan gradually learned to get more in touch with his feelings.

Edward was a bank manager who had to take early retirement after a nervous breakdown. A high-principled and intelligent man, he had joined the bank with the desire to serve and help people, and had done very well until aggressive new business techniques were introduced. He found himself in the position of having to persuade people to take on commitments that he knew they could not afford, which went against all his ideals and instincts. The situation was made worse by clashes with his immediate superior, a man he found unsympathetic and harsh. At this point, the bank situation began to stir up immensely painful memories from the past, which Edward had managed to bury for over thirty years. The encounters with his superior recalled the terrifying interrogations that Edward had suffered at the hands of his father, a brutal bully who had sexually abused Edward's two sisters and wrecked Edward's confidence in himself. Confronted with his long-buried feelings, Edward found that his rage, hatred, and despair were almost intolerable. His usual way of solving problems by intellectual reasoning was useless, and he could only find temporary respite by going on long solitary cycle rides. As he walked round the well-to-do suburb where he lived, which he described as an 'enclave of bank managers', he was greeted enviously by former colleagues who told him how lucky he was to be out of the rat-race. This was small comfort to Edward, who since the loss of his job had felt ostracized from society, a man with no contribution to make and no purpose to his life.

Finally, here is an example of a man who, as the result of being brutalized in his early childhood, cut himself off from his own feminine side and created a caricature of the macho man. But his inability to come to terms with his feminine aspects was reflected in his obsession with and hatred for women, which he eventually took to its logical extreme:

The macho man consumed by hatred for women — *Daily Express* headline 6 November 1986.

M4 rapist John Steed created a macho-man image which girls found irresistible — but behind the façade lay a dark secret. Steed hated women and enjoyed sex only when holding a victim at the point of a knife or the barrel of a gun. Steed, a physical fitness fan, built up his muscles during endless weight-lifting sessions. He loved driving fast cars, which he stole to impress women. His screen idol was the rough detective Dirty Harry, played by Clint Eastwood. 'He could never have any human relationships', said 45-year-old Sheila Steed (his mother). 'Even as a toddler he could never let anyone cuddle him. His father used to beat him, and I remember on his first day at school he went off without as much as a goodbye.'

The painful conflicts that arise when male sex role expectations clash with female ones form the background to just about every problem that arises in marital therapy, and indeed in male/female relationships in general. It can be very dispiriting for a therapist to watch the same issues coming up time after time, over and over again, with couple after couple, and to ponder on the amount of collective misery that these arguments represent across the country. Here are some highly typical examples:

She is upset. In fact she has been upset for some time and waiting for him to notice, but he has not. Eventually she starts to cry. He at once feels very uneasy. Probably this is because her display of emotion threatens to trigger off his own buried feelings, although he is not consciously aware of this. He volunteers an instant solution, 'Don't cry now', 'There's no point thinking about that', or 'I'll make you a cup of tea'. She senses that he is trying to put the lid on her feelings when what she really wants is not an instant answer, but for him to just sit with her and listen and understand. She either feels very confused because her feelings have been discounted, or gets even more upset at his lack of understanding. He can't stand this escalation of emotion and escapes by walking out of the room, leaving her feeling even worse than before.

He is upset and withdraws into himself. She can sense that there is something wrong and wants to know what it is and help, but she can't get him to admit or say what's really on his mind. He can't understand why she won't leave him alone to deal with the problem on his own. He thinks that all this talking she is so keen on will just make the whole thing worse. At a deeper level, he is very scared of stirring up feelings he can't handle. He withdraws even more, and she, frustrated at being shut out of his inner world, pursues him. He yells at her to stop nagging and give him some peace. Now she is upset too, and he feels ashamed and guilty, but unable to admit that either. Later he goes out to the pub and calms himself with a pint and a soothing and impersonal talk with his mates.

She is at the end of her tether after a day of chores and screaming kids. She is cross at the prospect of yet another chore, the evening meal, and wants him to offer to help, but can't ask him directly. This is partly because she sees it as basically her job, partly because she finds it hard to ask for anything anyway, and partly because she doesn't want to have to ask him — she wants him to realize how she feels without being told, just as she can sense how he feels. If he doesn't, it must be either deliberate obtuseness or a sign that he doesn't really care. She starts banging pans noisily. He now realizes something's wrong, and, lacking her skills as a mind-reader, wonders what the hell it is. Eventually she yells, 'Why can't you come and lend a hand for once?' 'Why on earth didn't you say so before, if that's what you want?', he yells back, and the 'reasonableness' of his reply infuriates her even further. He still can't work out exactly what he's done wrong, and mutters to himself about the illogical nature of women. He spends his whole life working to buy her washing machines and Hoovers and God knows what else — isn't that enough?

He can't understand why she has to make such a big issue of the housework. Sometimes he thinks she makes work for herself with all that unnecessary polishing and tidying. She's always on at him to stop leaving his clothes around and fix the bathroom door. He doesn't know quite why he hasn't got around to it yet, but none of these things are as important to him as to her — in fact, he doesn't really notice them. The house doesn't feel like his territory anyway: she chose the wallpaper and arranged the furniture and she spends the most time there. He feels more relaxed in the pub. He doesn't mind helping out with a bit of washing up or vacuuming, though. For her part, she can't make him understand that what gets her down is more than just the effort of shopping or dusting. It's the grind of doing the same tasks day after day and worst of all being responsible for them all the time, even if she works outside the home as well, so that she can never just assume that if she hasn't planned a meal, someone else will have thought to do something about it instead. She can't even trust him to load the washing machine on his own — last time, all the clothes came out pink. He knows it's not her job to do the DIY, so the least he could do would be to fix the bathroom door when she asks. It annoys her every time she sees it.

Let us return to the issue of how the psychiatric system deals with male role problems.

First, as we have seen, it can fail to recognize them, so that men who make up the other halves of women's problems are unhelped. Given the picture I have drawn of psychiatry so far, this might seem like a lucky escape. However, a good psychiatric service ought not to be colluding with the desire of some men to let their womenfolk bear their problems for them. In the end, the men lose out as well.

Second, there is the fact that medical model psychiatry is based on the belief that uncomfortable feelings, like the symptoms of an illness, should be suppressed and eliminated rather than expressed, worked through, and understood in relation to the rest of the person's life. The most obvious way to do the former is by prescribing pills. Well-meaning but unsophisticated staff acting on the same assumptions will try to cheer up any patient who looks unhappy and hustle them into discussion groups or other activities. Nurses feel they have to keep busy rather than be found 'just chatting' to the patients. This is damaging for both sexes, but for men it coincides particularly unfortunately with the messages of the male role which may be what led to their problems in the first place. Men who cannot express their feelings or who have hidden them with frantic activity or drugs like alcohol, may find that their treatment consists of learning new ways to distance themselves from their feelings and put the lid on their emotions. This may suit them in the short term; in fact, they may have come along asking for an instant solution in the form of a pill that takes the problem away so that they can carry on exactly as before. Unfortunately such remedies rarely work out. It is much more likely that they will need to return for more 'patching up' with medication and admission, which again only works for a while. For example, John, who needed to grieve for his dead father, had already had one admission to hospital after a previous bereavement and had been sent out again with a prescription; when he at last started to feel his grief, his doctors became alarmed and increased his medication.

More generally, the whole practice of psychiatry is based on traditionally masculine values. Psychiatrists strive very hard to present psychiatry as a legitimate and respectable branch of medical science, so that they can maintain their claim that the psychiatric service must be headed by doctors rather than, say, nurses or social workers or a team of professionals working as equals. This means that there is an overriding emphasis on diagnosing, labelling, and categorizing patients and prescribing medical-type solutions for their problems, rather than on a more 'feminine' exploring of feelings and relationships. The prime example of this is the *Diagnostic and Statistical Manual of Mental Disorders, Third Edition* (known as *DSM – III*),[21] the psychiatrist's guide to diagnosis, which in 472 pages labels and divides psychiatric problems into literally hundreds of sections and sub-sections in a manner which in a patient would be seen as a sign of obsessive-compulsive-disorder (*DSM – III* definition: 'repetitive and seemingly purposeful behaviours that are performed according to certain rules or in a stereotyped fashion'). The same attitude is evident in many psychiatric textbooks, which devote pages to the discussion of 'undifferentiated neuroses', 'relative frequency of common symptoms', 'differential diagnosis', 'biochemical and endocrine investigations', 'genetic factors and prognosis', while psychiatric journals carry articles with daunting titles like 'Information processing and attentional functioning in the developmental course of schizophrenic disorders', or, 'A controlled comparison of flupenthixol and amitriptyline in depressed out-patients', or 'Affective disorder: Is reactive depression an entity?', or 'Biochemical and pharmacological studies: The dopamine hypothesis', and so on. Researchers into schizophrenia have attempted to demonstrate differences in eye movements, skin conductance, pain perception, body temperature rhythm, attitudes towards 'body products', blood types, intake of wheat gluten, season of birth, production and judgement of humour, handwriting, body odour, finger ridge count, hand structure, femininity, composition of blood, hair, urine, and countless other variables.[22]

While all this may have its relevant aspects, what is so striking is the absence of the real person to whom all these diagnoses and hypotheses are attached; the disregard of relationship factors, so that psychiatric problems are assumed to be rooted in one person only; and the lack of any socioeconomic context to put it all in. Amidst all this important and scientific-sounding literature, the human reality of the lives of distressed men and women is in danger of getting lost altogether. Prestige in psychiatric circles is not generally gained by having an interest in psychotherapy and wide experience of helping people with relationship problems; indeed this may be a positive handicap. Psychiatrists rise to the top of their profession by research and publication in respectable, scientific, objective fields, and may be able to carve out a distinguished position for themselves while having no aptitude whatsoever for forming therapeutic relationships with their patients. The only other approach to have gained a firm foothold in psychiatry, behaviour therapy, is of a goal-oriented, symptom-removing nature.

Given the predominance of 'masculine' values, it is not surprising that psychotherapy, which requires that its clients (and its practitioners) are 'feminine' enough to ask for help, expose their vulnerable sides, acknowledge their feelings, allow themselves to depend on someone else, and suspend their desire for an instant clear-cut solution is regarded with suspicion, and may be downgraded as 'unproven' if it is available at all. All these requirements may be difficult for anyone, but are likely to be particularly hard for men, since they run directly contrary to the messages of the male role. I do not wish to present psychotherapy as an ideal answer to everyone's problems. For many people, social interventions, behavioural techniques, low-key support, or simply a rest and a break are what is needed most. Some psychotherapeutic approaches, particularly of the more psychoanalytic type, can degenerate into stale intellectualizing and word-games and are just as guilty as medical model psychiatry of taking responsibility away from people and fostering unhealthy dependence. It is an unfortunate fact that people tend to gravitate towards the therapies that suit them least. Men who already have a tendency to cut off their feelings and seek rational/intellectual solutions may need to be guided towards the newer therapies, such as Gestalt, which place greater emphasis on touch, intuition, and emotional expression.

We saw how female patients find few role-models of assertive, powerful women when they come into hospital. There is a corresponding problem for male patients, who are unlikely to come across many male staff, particularly high-status ones, who are comfortable enough with their feminine side to drop their professional front and admit to fears and vulnerabilities, who can be gentle, sensitive, and intuitive, and who are not ashamed even to hug or cry with their patients on occasion. The very idea seems bizarre and embarrassing. In fact, the underlying masculine ethos generally means that there is far more emphasis on competing than on caring in the higher ranks of the staff. When I first started to work in this field, my naive expectation that mental health professionals would know better than others how to get on together was quickly shattered. Every hospital that I have worked in has had its long-running feuds between senior staff, the themes of which are often *competition* — for beds, wards, office space, junior staff, and other forms of power and status. *Caring* for patients is a very low priority in this political in-fighting, if indeed it is a factor at all.

None of this is meant to imply that the more 'masculine' values and approaches are mistaken or useless. Medication, diagnosis, research, goal-oriented approaches, and so on are extremely valuable in their place, while a more passive listening role is completely inappropriate in some cases. Patients who adopt the sick role, for example, may need to have a very tough and assertive line taken with them, while as discussed in Chapter 3, the absence of a treatment contract with clearly defined goals has disastrous consequences. What is needed is a balance between traditionally 'masculine' and 'feminine' values and approaches. A lack of balance is as damaging in a whole system as it is in an individual person. At present, in psychiatric hospitals as in the wider world, it is the 'feminine' which is lacking and which must be restored if the psychiatric system is to be able to guide its patients, male or female, back to balance and healing.

Part Two

THE SYSTEM

7

The professionals and their training

One of the problems that arises in trying to describe the day-to-day practice of psychiatry to people outside the business is that they find it hard to understand how such obviously inappropriate treatment can be handed out, while commonsense attempts to help patients to talk and to understand their home situations are ignored. Indeed, not all psychiatry is of this nature. Even the most backward hospital has its share of dedicated workers doing an excellent job within the limitations imposed by the institution, while some places are able to attract good staff and provide a good service to the majority of their patients. Unfortunately, these are the exceptions; the rule is typified by the cases presented so far which are not in fact among the more extreme examples that could be found. (For instance, there is only one case of compulsory admission.) Yet the great majority of psychiatric staff are dedicated and hard-working people with a genuine wish to help the patients they are paid to care for. So how does it come about that the results are often so damaging? A partial answer is supplied by looking at the training that different mental health professionals receive, which, as I hope to show, actually makes them less rather than more able to help people in mental distress. Setting this in the context of a brief history of psychiatry and examining the role of the drug companies may provide further clues. First, though, it is time to look at the psychiatric system from the point of view of the professionals.

PSYCHIATRISTS

Psychiatrists are doctors who have followed the basic five- or six-year medical training and then chosen to specialize in psychiatry, rising up the medical hierarchy from Senior House Officer to Registrar, Senior Registrar and possibly, in the end, Consultant. Consultant psychiatrists are at the head of the traditional psychiatric team and wield a great deal of power politically, not being accountable to the new general managers who have been appointed to rationalize the health service, and in terms of patient care, where they make the ultimate decisions about treatment.

There is a common misconception of a psychiatrist as a bearded man who asks you to lie on a couch and free-associate about your dreams while he offers Freudian interpretations of your remarks. In fact, this is a more accurate description of a psychoanalyst in private practice. Psychiatrists are often, in the words of one of them,

> critical, sceptical, and even hostile to psychoanalysis and psychodynamics [and] have very little, or no use for them, either in their own theoretical and empirical enquiry or in their practical work. These psychiatrists appear to make up the . . . mainstream of the profession. In contrast, there are other psychiatrists, the minority of the profession apparently, who are favourably disposed to analysis and psychodynamics, and who do make use of them, to some degree at least, and in some way or ways.[1]

Junior psychiatrists arrive at their first jobs having had only eight weeks' exposure to psychiatry, and no training in counselling or psychotherapy, to be faced with a bewildering series of patients, many of whom are long-term attenders inherited from a succession of previous post-holders. They are expected to pick up the relevant skills on the job, and how successfully this occurs depends on the willingness of the consultant to offer supervision and support and their own enthusiasm for searching out extracurricular training courses and workshops. Having to move to a different post every six months does not help continuity of care for the patient or of learning experience for the doctor.

Psychiatrists' training and backgrounds do not necessarily equip them to understand the mixture of emotional distress and social deprivation that make up many patients' problems. Less than 3 per cent are drawn from unskilled or semi-skilled backgrounds.[2] Medical training, with its emphasis on physical facts, probably discourages more psychologically-minded candidates from entering the profession.

> Concentration on school-leaving attainment in science subjects may lead to negative selection as far as potential interest in psychiatry is concerned. The present restrictive entrance requirements . . . act to screen out school leavers who have the general interest in literature, philosophy and the arts which often accompanies what may broadly be called a psychological orientation.[3]

Once on the course, this emphasis is reinforced. Modern medicine values the scientific rather than the empathic approach, i.e. diagnosis and the prescribing of physical treatments rather than counselling and an understanding of psychological factors, although in recent years more social science has been introduced into the curriculum. Such psychotherapeutic input as there is tends to be of little practical use in day-to-day patient management, i.e. lectures on Freud rather than on commonsense basic counselling skills, while newer therapies such as Transactional Analysis and Gestalt are completely ignored.

Psychiatry is a very low-status speciality in medicine — seen as the least desirable after dermatology — and only 7 per cent of newly qualified doctors think of it as an attractive career.[4] Thus, many psychiatrists will have arrived in psychiatry through failure to get into their preferred speciality, rather than through a positive choice on their part. The lack of applicants has been the subject of several conferences, where some medical students pointed out that 'During the eight weeks that we are allotted to learn the subject there is little time to teach these special skills, the ability to deal with grief or anger, how to draw out patients and to develop a special relationship with them', and 'My contention is that if medical students are chosen from people brought up in the science A-levels, reinforcing them with a "learn-in, fact-a-day" type of medical training, they cannot be expected to be psychiatrists or to want to be psychiatrists.'[5]

The shortfall in applicants is made up by large numbers of overseas-trained doctors who fill about half of all posts, mostly in the lower grades, although the introduction of restrictions on immigration in 1985 is changing this situation to some extent. Some are excellent, but many are extremely poorly equipped for the job. As one psychiatrist writes,

It is clear that many doctors from overseas come here without any intention to take up the subject. They come here to obtain a higher qualification in medicine, surgery, or obstetrics, but because they have little money and are at a disadvantage when competing with home-trained graduates for the better training posts they have to be content with taking positions in less well-endowed hospitals, posts that British medical graduates would not touch under any circumstances.[6]

One writer describes the resulting dilemma:

Having chosen a field he is least interested to work in, befuddled by the terminology of dynamically-oriented psychiatry, perplexed by the anxiety-provoking interview of an acute admission ward, lacking fluency in the English language, let alone familiarity with the English culture and idiom, the postgraduate tries hard to put on a bold front.[7]

(Equally serious problems can arise when white doctors try to understand the difficulties of ethnic minorities — see Chapter 11.) Attracted from abroad with the promise of receiving post-graduate training, these doctors may find themselves forever stuck in the lower ranks of psychiatry while patient care inevitably suffers. The other group who, for different reasons, find it hard to move up the medical hierarchy are women who want to combine a career with a family. They often take up part-time posts as clinical assistants, but it is very difficult to move from there to a consultant post.

Traditional psychiatrists stick closely to the diagnosis-admission-and-medication routine, perhaps with some claims to be doing low-key supportive counselling as well. A minority of others, as we have seen from earlier chapters, attempt a more innovative approach. Many junior doctors in particular are very aware of the limitations of their training and are eager to fill the gaps if the opportunity presents itself.

PSYCHIATRIC NURSES

Psychiatric nurses follow a three-year training course, approximately six months of which is made up of formal teaching, the rest being spent in various placements. There is a mixture of medical input — anatomy, physiology, neurology and so on — and psychology and psychiatry.

Before the introduction of the 1982 syllabus, now in use almost everywhere, the training was much more closely based on general medicine, with the patient seen as someone suffering from a physically based illness which it was the nurses's job to cure by taking over from him or her and dispensing the correct medical treatment. There was very little emphasis on the nurse's own personal development, and though counselling was described as part of the treatment for some problems, it was not actually taught as part of the course.

The 1982 syllabus places greater emphasis on social factors, personal development, community work, and developing relationships with patients, and nurses are encouraged to draw up goals for their own group of patients. This is done according to the 'Nursing Process', a treatment-planning exercise derived from general medicine, in which problems are summarized under such headings as Needs/Problems, Intervention/Strategy, and Goal/Expected Outcome. Although it is essential to draw up a treatment plan for patients, a format which is suitable for physical illness (Problem: Patient has bed sores. Intervention: Turn the patient hourly. Expected outcome: Cure the bed sores, etc.) is not always so appropriate for emotional distress. Moreover, it is rarely integrated into the overall treatment policy laid down by the psychiatrists.

Although the importance of counselling is acknowledged, it is generally true that anything other than the most basic counselling skills have to be acquired after qualifying — if, that is, you can manage to get funding to go on the relevant courses. During their placements on the wards, low staffing levels often mean that student nurses have to be used as extra pairs of hands and thus miss out on supervision from trained staff.

Low pay and low status do not encourage recruits to any branch of nursing, and though there are many excellent nurses around, training courses cannot always afford to select out the less suitable candidates. Most newly-trained nurses are, of course, very young, and likely to be lacking in the life experience that would help them to understand their patients better. The position of a qualified nurse is in many ways very difficult. On the one hand, nursing can be a very safe and comfortable job once you have settled into the routine of an institution. On the other, short-staffing often makes it impossible to do more than keep up with basic paperwork and ward management, leaving little time for more satisfying and useful personal contact with the patients. In any case, nurses' contributions tend to be undervalued by other staff, by relatives who will ask to see 'the doctor' for preference, and by patients themselves, many of whom hold a strong faith in the magic words of the psychiatrist even if the latter has only been in psychiatry a matter of months as opposed to the nurse's several years. Close day-to-day contact with the long-term and readmission cases on whom everyone has given up induces a sense of failure. Nurses as a group are not good at speaking up for themselves, and in any case the rigid nursing hierarchy, where every move has to be approved by a series of seniors with the power of veto, makes it very hard to introduce changes. It is not surprising that demoralization, sometimes leading to a sense of resigned helplessness or to Persecutory attitudes towards patients, is widespread in the profession.

Community Psychiatric Nurses (CPNs) undergo an extra year of training, although this is not compulsory, and have established themselves, not without opposition, as a fairly independent profession. In many areas they receive direct referrals from GPs and can thus build up their own caseload and style of working away from the hospital, by basing themselves in clinics and surgeries and visiting patients in their homes.

Traditional nurses, some of whom still wear uniforms, stick mainly to carrying out the basic tasks of ward management, pill-dispensing, or, in the community, giving slow-release injections of medication. Others try to become more involved with ward groups, counselling individual patients, and seeing relatives, while in the community there may be considerable scope for developing their own interests in family therapy, group therapy, and other areas.

OCCUPATIONAL THERAPISTS

The three-year occupational therapy training course has, like nursing, a large medical input — anatomy, physiology, neurology, surgery — as well as covering basic psychology and sociology, and equips occupational therapists to work with the physically disabled or the mentally handicapped as well as with psychiatric patients. The emphasis is on helping people through practical activities such as shopping, cooking, handicrafts, work projects, discussion groups, and so on. Counselling and psychotherapy play very little part in the training course, although there are moves to change this. About half of the occupational therapy department in psychiatric hospitals is made up of occupational therapy helpers, untrained people with practical skills and an interest in psychiatry.

Occupational therapists can feel undervalued by doctors and other staff who use them merely to divert and occupy patients, and do not appreciate the contribution that they can make from their often very detailed first-hand knowledge of the patients and their difficulties. Traditional occupational therapists work very much in line with the psychiatrists' suggestions and confine themselves to a practical, problem-solving approach. Others see their role as a more independent and psychotherapeutic one in which individual, family, and group therapy also play an important part.

CLINICAL PSYCHOLOGISTS

This is a relatively new and small profession. Unlike psychiatrists, psychologists do not have a medical training and as a result they tend to hold rather different views about psychiatry. Clinical psychology is seen as a desirable option for psychology graduates and courses are heavily oversubscribed. Successful (and mostly middle-class) applicants follow their first degree in psychology with a two- or three-year training course consisting mainly of placements in hospitals and clinics. Carrying out therapy under supervision is a very important part of training, although some courses still insist that behaviour therapy is the only respectable approach, with other forms of psychotherapy being regarded with suspicion.

The main areas in which psychologists work are psychiatry, mental handicap, the prison service, with the elderly, and with children. Their position in psychiatric hospitals is rather ambiguous. On the one hand they do not have the power and influence of the psychiatrists, which can lead to very frustrating situations in in-patient work if patients are suddenly discharged or put on medication or transferred to another ward in the middle of a treatment plan. On the other hand, psychologists do not have the same rigid professional hierarchy as doctors and nurses, and since they can accept referrals directly from GPs, they can build up their own independent caseload and work fairly autonomously. Many psychologists choose to avoid the difficulties inherent in hospital-based work by doing this.

Traditionally, psychologists have special expertise in psychological testing (assessing IQ scores, brain damage, personality characteristics, and so on) and in research and behaviour therapy. In recent years psychologists have expanded their role to become involved in other fields instead or as well, for example, psychotherapy of various kinds with individuals, families, couples, and groups, training and supervising other staff, and developing new ways of giving a service such as holding sessions in GP surgeries and clinics.

SOCIAL WORKERS

All social workers follow a general training course, usually two years long, which qualifies them to work in a wide variety of settings: district teams, residential units, hostels, hospitals, probation, and so on. The course covers such areas as law and criminology, social policy, welfare rights, and work with the elderly and mentally handicapped as well as mental health, and students do projects and supervised placements (which take up about eight months of the course) in the area in which they wish to specialize. Practical training in basic counselling skills with individuals, families, and groups is also a standard part of the course.

The general orientation of social work courses is sociological and psychological rather than medical, and the emphasis is on understanding the client in his or her social context. Thus, there will be consideration of such issues as the influence of class, race, and gender, and of socioeconomic factors, and students will be expected to become involved not only with the clients themselves but with families and housing agencies, to help with financial problems and so on, and to know about local community facilities. Partly because of their training and partly because of the kind of people who are attracted to the job in the first place, social workers as a group tend to be less favourably disposed towards the use of physical treatments in psychiatry and more concerned with psychological and social interventions, democratic teamwork, and patients' rights. Although social work has a middle-class image, policies such as having special access courses for members of ethnic minorities and the educationally disadvantaged and placing importance on life experience, not merely on academic qualifications, mean that students come from a wider range of backgrounds than is found in some other mental health professions. The majority of entrants are women, although men are disproportionately represented in the higher ranks.

Most social workers in psychiatric hospitals will be involved in counselling and psychotherapy as part of their job. Family therapy is often a special interest. They operate fairly independently and have their own caseload. A psychiatrist who wants to have someone compulsorily detained in hospital has to obtain the agreement of an Approved Social Worker who has undergone a special course in the relevant mental health legislation.

PSYCHOTHERAPISTS

'Psychotherapist' is a general term for anyone who practises psychotherapy of any kind, whether they are doctors, nurses, social workers, or whatever. There are a very few posts in the NHS for 'Psychotherapist' or 'Consultant psychotherapist', and they are generally attached to teaching hospitals. They are usually filled by psychiatrists who have trained in psychotherapy for several years in addition to their medical training, and who tend to be very much influenced by psychoanalysis (i.e. in-depth individual therapy over several years). Studies claim to show that psychotherapy is best suited to the YAVIS client (Young, Attractive, Verbal, Intelligent and Successful — and, one might add, probably Female too). While this may merely be a reflection of psychotherapists' difficulty in understanding those who are not of their own class and kind, it is certainly true that the average psychiatric patient needs something a good deal more flexible, informal, and commonsense than in-depth individual analysis, with relatives and practical forms of help being involved as necessary. This means that even where psychotherapy is available on the NHS, it tends to operate as a sort of fringe benefit for articulate middle-class patients without having much influence on the general ethos of the hospital. The other patients, who may be neither young, nor particularly attractive, verbal, intelligent, or successful, are left to struggle on with the same old physical treatments as before.

ART THERAPISTS AND MUSIC THERAPISTS

These two new professions are still very small in numbers. People with a degree or diploma in art or music follow this with a postgraduate course (one year for art therapists, three years for music therapists) which teaches them to use these skills therapeutically with individuals and groups. The orientation is a non-medical psychotherapeutic one, with painting and music used as tools to reach, communicate with, and understand the whole person and their feelings.

GENERAL PRACTITIONERS

Although not part of the hospital-based psychiatric team, GPs have an extremely important role, since it is they who act as the gateway to psychiatric treatment by deciding whom to refer on, and equally importantly it is they who actually deal with the vast majority of mental health problems in the community. Psychological difficulties of various kinds make up perhaps the largest category of GP consultations, but one survey found that only 3.5 per cent of cases diagnosed as psychiatric by GPs were referred on to psychiatrists, with this decision being influenced as much by factors such as the patient's reluctance and the length of the waiting list as by the severity of the problem.[8] Most people with psychiatric problems, therefore, manage to get along somehow with the help of their GP, who, often knowing the patient and his/her family very well, tends to take a more commonsense view of mental distress than the psychiatrist. In fact in some psychiatric hospitals the GP trainees who pass through on placement are of a notably higher calibre than the doctors who are intending to make psychiatry their career.

GPs follow the basic 5 to 6 year medical training with two years of six-month placements in hospitals, which might or might not include a psychiatric hospital, according to choice, and one year as a trainee in a GP practice. Although courses, especially the newer ones, do include some counselling training, this is likely to be fairly elementary, and of course the 6 to 10 minutes allotted to each patient leaves very little time to go into problems in any depth. One result is a tendency to reach for the tranquillizer/anti-depressant as a quick solution, although there are some very good GPs around who do somehow manage to make time for a more psychological approach to patients in emotional distress.

It can be seen that in each profession, the more traditional staff tend to see themselves as members of a hierarchy with a definite but limited role which is primarily to do with diagnosing, testing, organizing, or doing practical medical or administrative tasks. The new-style staff, on the other hand, see themselves as operating more independently, and often in the face of considerable opposition have moved towards a broader and basically psychotherapeutic role with the traditional tasks of their profession being subordinate to this. Moreover, it is the most powerful (psychiatrists) and numerous (nurses) professions that receive the least psychotherapeutically-oriented training, so that such skills are most likely to be possessed by the newer, more peripheral, and less influential professions.

Of course, ward management, testing, diagnosis, and so on all have their value, but when these skills are not grounded in a psychotherapeutic understanding of people's feelings and relationships there is a danger that the whole person, whole system approach will be completely lost, with the kind of results that we have seen. The medically-based training of doctors and nurses in particular encourages them to override their natural commonsense reactions and see their charges as patients with illnesses, rather than people with problems. Not only are most mental health professionals not trained to see people in a whole-person, whole-system way, they are actually trained not to do so. All of this means that although each member of staff may be doing the best job they can within the limitations imposed by their own training and the institution itself, the results can still be disastrous.

Let us take as an example a hypothetical Mrs Smith, who is suffering from women's role problems; she is depressed, confused, not very assertive, and has never really questioned the belief that medical experts know what is best for her. Referred by her GP, she is first seen by a junior doctor who has only been in psychiatry for four months. He listens sympathetically and takes a detailed history, but when she says, 'I know I *ought* to be happy — why do I feel so depressed?' he has no more idea than she does, and nor does he know how to set about finding out. Still, she is distressed and he feels he has to do something. The safest and easiest option seems to be to make a diagnosis of 'Depression in a vulnerable personality', start her on some anti-depressants, and suggest that she comes into hospital 'for assessment', in the hope that this will give him more of an idea how to proceed. Mrs Smith is so desperate for help that it does not occur to her to refuse, although she is terrified at the idea of going into psychiatric hospital which to her (and her family) confirms that she must be crazy. Now officially labelled as the 'sick one', she arrives on the ward still not sure quite why she is there and what is going to happen to her, and the nurses, who are equally uninformed about the reason and purpose for her stay, show her around and assign her a bed.

A few days later there is a ward round, where representatives of all the staff meet to discuss the patients. As usual there is a long list and by the time Mrs Smith's name is reached, there are only five minutes left. The junior doctor explains to the consultant who has overall charge of her case that Mrs Smith is 42, was born and brought up in the area, is married with three children, works part-time in a shop, is in regular contact with her sister and mother who live nearby, has no previous psychiatric history although her paternal grandfather suffered from senile dementia, describes herself as having always been rather shy and anxious, and for the last three months has been feeling increasingly depressed, tearful, and unable to enjoy life or cope with her day-to-day chores. The consultant, who has no more training in a psychological understanding of depression than his junior, sees no reason to query the summary and diagnosis but suggests a change in the medication. He also asks a nurse to bring Mrs Smith into the room so that he can explain who he is, tell her that she will be staying for a few weeks so that the staff can get to know her better and try to help her, and ask her if she has any questions. Much too terrified to speak out in front of this circle of staring strangers, Mrs Smith says very little. This is the only time the consultant ever meets her.

In the absence of any coherent treatment plan, Mrs Smith has, unknown to her, been assigned to a standard package of activities in the occupational therapy department. The occupational therapists conscientiously arrange sessions of pottery and discussion groups for her. Since she is complaining of being unable to cope with the household chores, it seems a good idea to get her to do some cooking. If it turns out that she doesn't know how to cook they will be able to help, although if (as is almost certainly the case) she is perfectly competent but just feels panicky and hopeless at the thought of the chores, they will not know how to help her work out why this should be so. Meanwhile the nurses have drawn up a care plan for Mrs Smith, with various aims and strategies in addition to giving medication. For example, they believe that part of her problem is low self-esteem, and so they aim to praise and encourage her for any achievements during her stay. Noticing her anxiety, they are teaching her relaxation exercises. They also plan to allow her time to talk over her worries about her family. All this is fine as far as it goes except that it is not integrated into the rest of her treatment, so that anything that emerges during these talks is unlikely to be relayed to the consultant who makes the final decisions about Mrs Smith. Nor is it seen as part of the nurses' role to meet and do counselling work with Mrs Smith's husband and family, who are alarmed and confused about what is happening to her. In any case, there is little time for such meetings on an under-staffed ward. Lacking the training and information to work out how Mrs Smith's problems relate to the rest of her life and family, let alone how to help her with the restructuring of her role and attitudes that may be necessary, the nurses may fall back on well meaning reassurance and reminders of how lucky she is to have such a lovely family, which increase her guilt without helping her to understand herself any better.

After a few weeks, Mrs Smith is feeling no better. The things that were originally suggested as a way of working out what the treatment should be — admission to get to know her better, occupational therapy programmes to assess her practical abilities — have turned into the treatment itself. Mrs Smith continues to be an inpatient and to follow a standard programme of activities and outings because no one has the skills or knowledge to come up with a better plan, and she herself becomes increasingly desperate as her stay lengthens. A flavour of this reaches the ward round, where the consultant suggests several more changes in medication. A couple of other avenues are tried; the social worker is asked to sort out the Smiths' rent, and since Mrs Smith is complaining of forgetfulness, it seems a good idea to ask the psychologist to assess her memory and do some personality tests. The referral is in fact a covert plea for some suggestion as to how to deal with this puzzling woman, but the psychologist either does not realize this or does not see it as her job to do more than respond to the particular question that has been asked. She therefore does the tests and reports back to the consultant that Mrs Smith's memory is fine but that she has very low self-esteem and a tendency to internalize her anger. No one reports this back to Mrs Smith, who remains puzzled by the whole episode, and nor does anyone have any clear idea how to incorporate this information into a treatment plan although it is dutifully added to Mrs Smith's medical notes.

The pattern is set for heavier measures to be tried — ECT perhaps. The longer Mrs Smith stays in hospital the worse she feels, and the less able she is to face the home situation she came from. Side-effects from the medication add to her misery, and since she has not been warned about them she takes them as further evidence of mental illness. By now both she and her family see her as pretty sick, but this leads them all to the conclusion that she needs more hospital treatment, not less. She is set to follow the same path as Elaine or Mary. And yet none of this has come about through any deliberate unkindness or neglect on the part of the staff, each of whom has only been doing their job, albeit along rather traditional and unimaginative lines.

The argument is clear: that the hospital will be able to offer real help and healing only to the extent that it is able to move away from the divided function, medical model approach to one where a psychotherapeutic, whole-person, whole-system understanding of people's problems underlies the training of all the different professions, and the promotion of this approach is seen as everyone's role and resonsibility. This raises the important question of how, if it is so unhelpful, the underlying medical model philosophy has come to exert such a powerful influence on the training of mental health professionals. To answer this we need to look briefly at the history of psychiatry over the last 200 years. Meanwhile we can end this chapter by hearing from two hospital workers whose contributions are usually overlooked but who, unhandicapped by a professional training, often have refreshingly straightforward views on the whole situation. First, a woman who has worked in the administrative and clerical department of a psychiatric hospital for ten years:

I think we have an important part to play. We will help the

patients sort out their rent, gas, electricity. You can't help but become involved with the patients. We have some that'll come in and talk to you — they usually come in for change, that's the excuse, and then they'll chat. Yes, you can start to be almost doing counselling. I think you are aware that you're not supposed to, but you do do it. The patient can put on a front to the doctor, and give a totally different picture when they come to us. Now you often get the ward concerned about so-and-so's language or so-and-so's behaviour. Now I find it interesting that we don't get that in the office. We very rarely have a scene in the office, because we've got the money, it's as simple as that, and again it depends on how important their money is to them. I think as well they're always in a one-to-one situation with us, they're not in the ward with the nurses all running round busy, they're getting that attention.

Money is a big part of their problems. If you've got no money it's hard to cope, isn't it. It makes a change if someone comes in here and says they're working. It's especially bad if they're, say, 40 to 60 and they've got little chance of finding another job, so leaving aside the money aspect they've lost their self-respect, they feel useless. There are people who come in who are comfortably off, no, not a lot of them, but a minority. The majority I would think are from [naming the poorer areas of town]. Some of them are ill, some of them you wonder why they're staying, some you think they've been here far too long, and some you know we'll become a crutch to and they'll come back. The readmission figures show that. Three patients came in to visit last night after 5 o'clock. Now who were they visiting? I daresay they found somebody. They might say, 'I just want to see if anyone I know is in', and you haven't got the heart to say no, maybe there you've got someone who's asking for help again. I don't know what you can do about it at this stage — it should have been done before, they shouldn't have been kept in this long in the first place.

Sometimes you wonder if the relatives should be in instead of the patient. Sometimes you wonder if the relative has *put* the patient in! I find it interesting on sections [i.e. compulsory admissions] that applications are done by social workers, and it's very very rare, we've only had one, where a relative will do the application, and by that I see that the relative is feeling guilty if someone is being put on section, but they don't mind the social worker doing it and bringing the patient into

167

hospital. Should we be looking more at families? By having family groups and bringing the mother and father and sister and brother in, I think that would help enormously. We've got an example now, haven't we, Elizabeth Black [a 23-year-old diagnosed as schizophrenic] — now her mother drives Elizabeth mad! Elizabeth can be quite happy, she'll come in and she'll chat and she's all right, and then mother appears on the scene. You know, mother will say to us, 'Are you going to talk to her, about the way she's spending her money?'. It's Elizabeth's business how she spends her money. But her mother goes on and on, and when she appears she causes such a fuss. She agitates her. But this happens with quite a few of them. Again, the professionals should be seeing the families. We [the administrative staff] can't do anything really — we can listen, but I would worry about us listening too much and where the cut-off point is. I would think a lot of the families should be seen because no matter what you do for that patient in here, when you're going to put them back in the same environment they came from, surely they're going to go under again. And then maybe the relative would start to get some understanding of it. Or some understanding of themselves. I think it's obvious they don't know — I mean, not for a minute would Elizabeth's mother see herself as hurting Elizabeth — she loves the girl.

I've got very mixed feelings about the staff. We've got some very good ones and we've got some poor ones that I would watch like a hawk. We've got a couple that would make me worry about abuse — hitting patients. Some of the doctors are super. But others — I don't know how we get these people who can barely speak English in a psychiatric unit, where it's not about cutting anybody up, it's about talking. Well, how the devil are they going to talk? It's not doing the patient any good, and I'm sure it's not doing the doctor any good. We've had some you don't even know what they're talking about and some who were very caring. No, I wouldn't speak out about these things. I think I'd be told somewhere along the line that we're not professionals.

A woman who has worked in the medical records department of a psychiatric hospital for eight years is more outspoken:

Each patient has to be judged differently really. You get some that come in and they're very ill, and they don't even know what day it is, but then quite often the relatives fetch them in and you're asking them questions and the relatives are answering for them and they haven't got a chance really because they've decided the patient's ill and that's it. But I think you've got to let the patients speak otherwise they're just nothing, they just sit there and let somebody speak for them all the time. You see it all here — it's like watching a play sometimes. You definitely get a different picture from the doctors. Especially when you're on reception, I've heard patients saying on a Friday — Friday used to be discharge day — 'You just tell doctor so-and-so that you don't want to be discharged and that if he discharges you you know you're going to do something silly' — and they're priming each other up. But then let's face it, you come in here and you get company and food and your money sorted out, now do you want to go out there and live in a scruffy hotel room or a grotty council flat in a high rise or whatever, and all the loneliness? We've got the one lot that runs out and wants to discharge themselves, and the other lot that gets quite comfy thank you and doesn't want to go out and face up to their problems. But the longer you leave it, the bigger the problem, because they're getting more entrenched all the time, aren't they? We've had a couple of really good GP trainees in the past, and they've stood in the corridor and said, 'Out!' but I mean you get the waffly ones and they're dead scared to commit themselves and they're usually the ones that are going into psychiatry. But you've got to have the courage of your convictions if you're going to be in the psychiatric world. Because I mean this place would be packed to the gunnels if you didn't throw a few out now and again, wouldn't it? We've had some terrific doctors here, some really down-to-earth ones, but I think psychiatrists get too wound up in their own theories, and I think they sort of lose touch with what's ordinary. In their own home lives, obviously, most of them mix with medical people. But it's all right for me to sit and talk, but what happens if you put that patient out in the street and they go and throw themselves off the motorway bridge? I don't have the responsibility that the doctors have.

I've always taken it that mental health was an on-going thing, it's a very long-term thing. Schizophrenia is a recurring thing, isn't it? It's a very convenient label actually, isn't it, when in doubt put schizophrenia, but that's just my opinion which is an unqualified one. Now look at the alcoholics they take in here. It's a big farce isn't it, it really is. If you're alcoholic, nine-tenths of them are men or women who've been abandoned by their families because they are alcoholic, or even if they live with their families, they're not wanted. Now can you tell me what use it is bringing them in for a few weeks and drying them out? When they go out, where are their friends, where are the people that'll listen to them? In the pub. They're not going to go down there and start drinking orange juice all of a sudden, are they? They come up here with a letter from their GP and you open it and it says, 'This man would like to dry out and try and control his alcoholism' and they're standing there at 10 a.m. absolutely stinking to high heaven of alcohol for God's sake! But they still admit them don't they, and they walk out and go up the road to the bloomin' pub while they're here too. Waste of NHS money that is. No, I don't think that's the answer. I thought it was a terrific idea a while back when they were discussing this scheme, instead of bringing them straight into hospital a doctor and nurse went out to the patient's home and tried to sort out the patient's problems there. I thought that was really sensible, because you bring them in here and then you keep them in for a few days and send them out to their problems at home, and that's your readmission case that's going to keep coming back again. If they're kept in that situation with people to visit them, they're far more likely to stay out there and try to grapple with whatever's wrong. But it didn't come to anything. The only drawback to this place is that you only see the ones that keep coming back and don't get cured.

It is interesting to note that these members of staff may be doing as much or more counselling (unacknowledged) as the professionals, and may even be able and prepared to do things that the professionals back away from, challenging family interactions, for example. Domestics, too, often play a crucial but unacknowledged role in the ward culture. This is not to deny the value of expert skills, but to point out that the kind of training that many mental health professionals receive is not useful or appropriate to their task. In fact it has the effect of undermining whatever simple human warmth and understanding they started off with — qualities that can achieve a great deal on their own —

while acquiring psychotherapeutic skills actually requires professionals to unlearn the more medical aspects of their training.

Another interesting point is that much of what these two women are suggesting — meeting the relatives, visiting the home to see what the problem is, not letting people use the hospital just to escape their problems, supporting people when they leave hospital — could be dressed up in jargon as a plea for family therapy, crisis intervention teams, treatment contracts, and community care programmes. Basically, it is plain common sense. However they correctly believe that if they expressed such opinions openly, they would quickly be told that their lack of professional training disqualified them from passing judgement on such matters.

8

A brief history of psychiatry

The conventional account of the history of British psychiatry goes something like this: Despite some ups and downs and false starts, there has been slow but steady progress from the unenlightened days when lunatics were untreated or even tortured in places like Bedlam for the amusement of the public, to the present state of medical expertise. During the nineteenth century there was a gradual shift from a primitive view of madness as caused by supernatural agencies, to a more sophisticated medical view, with psychiatry becoming accepted as a standard part of medical training. The era of 'moral treatment', under the influence of Pinel in France and the Tukes in England, ended some of the worst excesses of the early attempts to treat madness, although unfortunately not all the old habits were eradicated, since the new asylums built in every county quickly became overcrowded. More liberal policies in the 1930s encouraged the setting up of local outpatient clinics and aftercare facilities for former patients, and the mood of optimism was increased by the discovery of new treatments such as insulin coma therapy (no longer used) and ECT. The 'drug revolution' of the 1950s, when several new classes of drugs were synthesized, enabled many of the most disturbed patients to be discharged into the community, or at least to spend long periods outside hospital, and the number of patients in psychiatric hospitals fell accordingly. Psychiatry is now accepted as just another branch of medicine, and patients can avoid much of the stigma associated with the old asylums by attending psychiatric units attached to district general hospitals. Of course, much still remains to be done; 'progress in this branch of medicine has been slow, but the difficulties to be contended with — professional apathy, public prejudice and the inherent complexity of the subject — have been very great',[1] but psychiatry can rightly be proud of its achievements to date. 'The treatment of psychosis, neurosis and schizophrenia have been entirely changed by the drug revolution. People go into hospital with mental disorders and they are cured' (Sir Keith Joseph introducing the 1971 White Paper, *Hospital Services for the Mentally Ill*).

Some such summary appears at the start of most standard textbooks on psychiatry. The alternative and far more controversial account is presented by writers such as Andrew Scull, who in his closely researched book *Museums of Madness* argues that to regard nineteenth-century lunacy reform as 'a triumphant and unproblematic expression of humanitarian concern is to adopt a perspective which is hopelessly biased and inaccurate: one which relies, of necessity, on a systematic neglect and distortion of the available evidence'.[2] He presents a rather less reassuring picture of the history of early psychiatry in terms of the medical lobby's struggle for power and control of the field.

AN ALTERNATIVE ACCOUNT

For most of the eighteenth century the first madhouses were run privately by people from many different backgrounds — the clergy, and other less respectable individuals hoping to make money out of the business. It was widely believed that madness was caused by witchcraft, or sinful behaviour. Scull describes how, seeking to enter this profitable field themselves, the medical profession, which up till now had taken very little interest in insanity, began to claim that it was a disease like any other for which the usual remedies of purges, vomits, bleedings, and coloured powders, which of course only they could administer, were the cure. Many were highly respected medical men, and since recovery seemed to occur spontaneously in about one-third of cases anyway, doctors were able to claim success for treatments which were not really any more effective than anyone else's.

Throughout the nineteenth century the doctors manoeuvred to gain acceptance for their views on madness and to control the way it was treated. Given their lack of genuine expertise on insanity, this was a difficult task. The most serious obstacle was the growth of what was called 'moral treatment', which was developed by a layman, William Tuke, and his colleagues at an asylum in York. The word 'moral' meant something equivalent to 'emotional' or 'psychological', and implied a compassionate and understanding approach to sufferers from mental distress. Tuke had investigated the various remedies recommended by the medical profession, which included bleeding, blisters, evacuants, and medicines of all kinds, and found that all were either useless or positively harmful, with the possible exception of warm baths for melancholics. From then on, the visiting physicians at York only attended to bodily illness, while the lay people who were in charge of the day-to-day running of the institution developed a new approach in place of the harsh physical remedies. Lunatics were seen as essentially human, although distressed, and in need of kind and respectful management and cheerful and homely surroundings.

Externally imposed medical remedies like purges and physical restraint had no place in helping lunatics regain their dignity and self-control. They were to be treated as far as possible as if they were in full possession of their wits, with the firm and confident expectation that they could return to more acceptable behaviour. This, for the Victorians, meant re-education in the socially approved virtues of industry, self-control, moderation, and piety. Patients were expected to conduct themselves respectably at the regular lunatics' balls, and to work diligently in the kitchens, the bakery, the gardens, and the hospital farms. The recovery of women in particular was defined in terms of their willingness to undertake cleaning, sewing, and laundry in a spirit of decorum and obedience. Nevertheless, this regime was undoubtedly more humane than the previous one, and many recoveries were reported. Its fame spread, and one physician wrote,

The . . . Quakers have demonstrated beyond contradiction, the very great advantages resulting from a mode of treatment in cases of Insanity much more mild than was before introduced into any Lunatic Asylum at home or abroad. In the management of this institution, they have set an example which claims the imitation, and deserves the thanks, of every sect and every nation.[3]

Not surprisingly, this view was not shared by most of his colleagues, whose claims to possess special skills in the treatment of the insane were being threatened. Prominent doctors responded with such assertions as 'The disease of insanity in all its shades and varieties, belongs, in point of treatment, to the department of the physician alone . . . the medical treatment . . . is that part on which the whole success of the cure lies',[4] and, 'Direct medical remedies can never be too early intoduced or too readily applied'.[5]

Indeed, the doctors had a very difficult task reasserting their authority in the face of a popular approach based on the whole idea that common sense and humanity, which any lay person might possess, were the curative factors. The exponents of moral treatment who took over the York Asylum from Dr Best, one of the most famous medical experts of the time, could hardly have been less flattering about the events of his reign. One of them, a magistrate called Higgins, pointed out that after Dr Best's departure the number of patient deaths per year fell from 20 to 4. He observed scathingly that

> amongst much medical nonsense, published by physicians interested to conceal their neglect, and the abuses of their establishments, it has been said, that persons afflicted with insanity are more liable than others to mortification of their extremities. Nothing of the kind was ever experienced at the institution of the Quakers. If members of the royal and learned College of Physicians were chained, or shut up naked, on straw saturated with urine and excrement, with a scanty allowance of food — exposed to the indecency of a northern climate, in cells having windows unglazed — I have no doubt that they would soon exhibit as strong a tendency to mortified extremities, as any of their patients.[6]

There was concern that

> the management of the insane has been in too few hands; and many of those who have been engaged in it, finding it a very lucrative concern, have wished to involve it in mystery, and, in order to prevent institutions for their cure from becoming more general, were desirous that it should be thought that there was some secret in the way of medicine for the cure, not easily found out.[7]

This in fact was written by a doctor, who recommended that the best safeguard against future abuses was to ensure that the care of the insane was not left to any one group of experts, medical or otherwise, but that asylums should be constantly supervised by lay people. Or, as Higgins remarked sarcastically, 'Who after this will doubt the efficacy of my medicine — visitors and committees? I will warrant it superior even to Dr Hunter's famous secret insane powders — either green or grey — or his patent Brazil salts into the bargain'.[8]

So, having failed to oust the new regime, those doctors who found their position threatened by it had to find some way of turning it to their advantage. An approach specifically developed to be carried out by lay people did not seem a very promising place to start. But Scull shows how the very open-mindedness of moral treatment, and the honesty and modesty of its claims, made it vulnerable to takeover bids by the medical profession. Tuke and his followers had not protected their position in the traditional way by forming organized groups of lay therapists with special training or entry qualifications. At the same time they openly admitted that 'as we . . . profess to do little more than assist Nature, in the performance of her own cure, the term *recovered*, is adopted in preference to that of *cured*'.[9] This left a gap into which the medical men could step with claims (however unfounded) of new remedies which really *did* cure insanity. At the same time they revived the use of cathartics and tried to take over the administration of warm baths to melancholics, arguing that such techniques were by no means 'of so simple and straightforward a nature as might be at first sight conceived' and really needed to be supervised by medically trained professionals. Something that worked to their advantage was the fact that Tuke and his colleagues, although rejecting medical remedies, had still kept to much of the actual language of medicine — 'patient', 'treatment', 'cure', and so on — which implied an illness model.

By the early nineteenth century, the doctors had gained enough ground to win an important battle and to deal the reform movement a serious blow. They successfully argued against legislation that would mean madhouses were under the strict supervision and control of a board of lay people, who would have the power to investigate patients' treatment, forbid harsh practices, and order any patient they considered sane to be discharged. Doctors insisted that only medical experts could undertake this task satisfactorily, and consolidated their victory with a spate of medical articles and complicated lists of diagnoses. Around this time, lectures on the treatment of insanity became part of the normal medical training. Moral treatment was too widely known and highly regarded to be dismissed, but the doctors were now in a position to propose a compromise which at first sight seemed very reasonable. Both moral and medical methods had something to offer, indeed a knowledge of moral treatment was an important part of a doctor's expertise, but the best results could be obtained by using a combination of both approaches. What this did, in fact, was reduce the status of moral treatment from a whole philosophy of care to a mere collection of techniques, while the doctor, as the only one who understood both approaches, was left firmly in charge of the whole enterprise. Towards the second half of the eighteenth century the first medical journals appeared, devoted to the theme that 'Insanity is purely a disease of the brain. The physician is now the responsible guardian of the lunatic and must ever remain so'.[10]

Of course, this still left the doctors with the big problem of actually demonstrating that there was a physical basis for mental illness, but despite their confident assertions that this was the case, no proof was forthcoming. This did not stop them from applying all sorts of bizarre and unpleasant physical treatments; in fact they did so with all the more enthusiasm, hoping to find successful remedies to back up their claim to have special skills and expertise. At various times, these remedies included 'hypodermic injections of morphia, the administrations of the bromides, chloral hydrate, hypocymine, physotigma, cannabis indica, amyl nitrate, conium, digitalis, ergot, pilocarpine',[11] thirty-four different emetics, and fifty different purgatives, sudden immersion in cold water or pouring 10 to 50 buckets of icy water on patients' heads, anointing shaven heads with vinegar, or raising blisters on the head and neck and rubbing salves into the pustules, applying ants or leeches to the skin, whipping with stinging nettles, making incisions in the skin, applying red hot pokers simultaneously to the head and the soles of the feet, drilling holes in the scalp, putting patients in revolving chairs that could be rotated so fast 'that a healthy, rational man would lose everything in his stomach in five minutes', applying restraining masks to the face, putting patients on a treadmill for up to forty-eight hours, ordering baths in thin gruel, milk or even gravy,[12] and many other even more bizarre devices. But although there was no shortage of theories to explain how these remedies were supposed to work (icy water was said to cool heads that had been made feverish by congestion of the blood, while emetics were justified by the belief that there was a close link between insanity and abdominal disorders) the proportion of recoveries to admissions remained distressingly low.

By now it was very obvious that these methods were not producing cures. This would have been more of a threat to the medical profession's position and claims with regard to insanity if the asylums had not, by this time, become so extremely useful to the communities they served. Any troublesome person could be sent there, whether insane, or old, infirm, poor, delinquent, simple-minded, or simply inconvenient to their families and neighbours. The inmates were in no position to complain, and the local officials found the arrangement too useful to worry very much about the validity of the doctors' claims to have special skills, although it was nice to be able to reassure oneself that sending people to the asylum was really in their best interests too. Meanwhile the asylums grew . . . and grew . . . and grew. The 1845 Lunatic Asylums Act made it obligatory for every county and borough in England and Wales to provide enough asylum space to serve the local population, but however big an asylum was planned, it never had enough space for the increasing number of so-called lunatics. The huge, forbidding Victorian buildings, more like small towns than hospitals with their chapels and farms, sometimes had over 2,000 inmates. Very few of them ever left the walls of these grim asylums again. The disappearance of the ideals of moral treatment was visible in the architecture: 'the wards are long, narrow, gloomy and comfortless, the staircases cramped and cold, the corridors oppressive, the atmosphere of the space dingy, the halls huge and cheerless. The airing-courts, although in some instances carefully planted, are uninviting and prison-like'.[13] (These places are still in use today, where they harbour a smaller but similar population of chronic cases.)

Since by now, as one asylum superintendent notes, 'it is totally impossible there to do more than know [the inmates] by name', it became increasingly difficult to maintain the fiction that such 'treatments' as cold water shocks and tranquillizing drugs were being used for therapeutic reasons, rather than merely to control and discipline the inmates. Depriving them of tobacco and recreation and keeping them on starvation diets also helped to maintain order. But there was one advantage to the increased numbers; doctors could now claim that their enormous workload prevented them from achieving the cures that were really within their power, although at the same time they firmly resisted the appointment of lay administrators to free them to give more attention to their patients.

DEVELOPMENTS IN PHYSICAL TREATMENTS

There is not enough space to describe in detail the subsequent history of psychiatry, during which the medical profession has continued to consolidate its monopoly over the treatment of the mentally distressed. A highlight was the discovery around 1900 that syphilis was the cause of general paralysis of the insane, which affected a large group of patients, and seemed to give hope that a physical basis would soon be found for all the other types of mental distress. This has yet to happen, but, as before, this has encouraged rather than diminished the search for effective physical treatments. In the 1930s, three new remedies were seized upon with enthusiasm. They were:

Insulin coma therapy

As well as controlling diabetes, insulin was thought to have a calming effect on psychotic patients. It was believed that the best results were obtained by using extremely high doses which put schizophrenic patients into life-threatening 30- to 50-hour comas, closely supervised by trained staff in special units. Magical results were claimed. It was not until twenty years later, by which time it was widely used, that a thorough study showed that the insulin itself had no therapeutic effect at all,[14] and that any improvements had to be attributable to the attention and excitement surrounding the treatment rather than to the treatment itself.

Electric shock treatment (also called electro-convulsive therapy or ECT)

The dramatic claims made for insulin coma therapy were

179

subsequently attached to ECT, still very widely used today. Electricity was used intermittently throughout the early history of psychiatry, for example, by John Wesley in the eighteenth century, who declared that from his shock machine 'hundreds, perhaps thousands, have received unspeakable good'.[15] In the 1930s it was revived on the basis of an inaccurate belief that schizophrenia and epilepsy never occur together and must be incompatible diseases, and that therefore drug-induced convulsions might help to cure schizophrenia. Unfortunately for the patients, the seizures were often violent enough to fracture spine, ribs, and limbs. Later, epileptic-type seizures were induced by passing an electrical current through the head, while a drug which causes temporary paralysis prevented bones being broken. The following rather chilling account describes how Cerletti and Bini, the Italian inventors of ECT, administered it for the very first time to a tramp found gibbering incoherently in a Rome railway station:

> He started to sing abruptly at the top of his voice, then he quieted down. . . . It was quite evident to all of us that we had been using a too low voltage. It was proposed that we should allow this patient to have some rest and repeat the experiment the next day. All at once the patient, who evidently had been following our conversation, said clearly and solemnly without his usual gibberish: 'Not another one! It's murder!' I confess that such explicit admonition under such circumstances, and so emphatic and commanding, coming from a person whose enigmatic jargon had until then been very difficult to understand, shook my determination to carry on with the experiment. But it was just this fear of yielding to a superstitious notion that caused me to make up my mind. The electrodes were applied again and a 110-volt discharge was applied for 1.5 seconds. We observed the same instantaneous brief, generalized spasm, and soon after, the onset of the classic epileptic convulsion. We were all breathless during the tonic phase of the attack, and really overwhelmed during the apnea as we watched the cadaverous cyanosis of the patient's face. . . . Finally, with the first stertorous breathing and the first clonic spasm, the blood flowed better not only in the patient's vessels but also in our own. . . . He rose to sitting position and looked at us, calm and smiling, as though to inquire what we wanted of him. We asked: 'What happened to you?' He answered:

'I don't know. Maybe I was asleep.' Thus occurred the first electrically produced convulsion in man, which I at once named electroshock.[16]

ECT is now described as the treatment of choice for severe depression. A muscle relaxant and an anaesthetic are always administered, unlike in the early days of its use, so that patients should suffer a minimum of discomfort.

Psychosurgery

Finally, and occasionally used today, there is psychosurgery. In its more primitive form a lobotomy or leucotomy involved the removal or destruction of nerve fibres in the frontal lobe of the brain in an operation known as the 'standard leucotomy'. This involved

> making a burr hole in the side of the head, above and in front of the ear, inserting a cutting instrument, sweeping it in an arc ... and thereby dividing as much white matter as possible. The same procedure was then repeated on the opposite side of the head. This operation was extremely crude in that at postmortem there was found to be extreme variation in the positioning of the cuts.[17]

The technique was later refined, although given the complexity of the brain and our limited knowledge about its functioning, it is still impossible to be at all precise about the effects one wishes to achieve.

As with every new technique, psychosurgery was initially hailed as a wonder treatment, and was used with enthusiasm on patients with a wide variety of problems: schizophrenia, depression, anxiety, phobias, personality disorders, and so on. Despite early claims of success, it became clear that there are many undesirable after-effects, including seizures, aggressiveness, and other undesirable personality changes, intellectual impairment, a general emotional blunting sometimes dubbed 'zombie-ism', and even death. More unusual after-effects were suffered by Moniz, the Portuguese neurologist credited with the invention of psychosurgery. Not only was he awarded the Nobel Prize for this innovation, but one of his leucotomized patients, presumably not so impressed by his achievements, put an end to his career by shooting him in the spine. Leucotomy is now restricted to the very occasional case where someone suffers from severe obsessional neurosis or is a serious management problem. No figures are available for the number of such operations performed — one estimate is 200 a year.[18] Whether or not it can actually claim to be offering a cure in any sense (if you removed the whole brain, would that be a complete cure?) is open to question, although its supporters would argue that in very severe suffering it is a valid option.

All these innovations were overshadowed by the most recent development, the 'drug revolution' of the 1950s and 1960s.

THE DRUG REVOLUTION

Drugs of various types have been used in psychiatry since the nineteenth century, but in the 1950s and 1960s several new classes of drugs were developed and became the basic tools of modern psychiatry. They are known under two different names, the generic name and the brand name, the latter being the same basic product marketed and packaged by a particular drug company. Since 1985 many brand name drugs are no longer available on the NHS, and the cheaper generic version is prescribed instead.

The new drugs are:

1. The neuroleptics, also known as *major tranquillizers*. As the name suggests, these have a very powerful sedative effect, and are mainly used on patients who are thought to have a psychotic illness such as schizophrenia.

2. *The anti-depressants*, of which there are two main types. The monoamine oxidase inhibitors or MAOIs are less frequently prescribed because they interact dangerously with certain foods like cheese, chocolate, and bananas. The other main group is the trycyclics.

3. *Lithium* is a simple salt that does not fit into any of the above categories, but is thought to be very effective in controlling manic-depressive disorders.

4. The benzodiazepines, also known as *minor tranquillizers*. These drugs are mostly used to relieve panic and anxiety, although some are used as sleeping pills.

The major tranquillizer chlorpromazine was developed first, by a French pharmaceutical (drug) company. The company that originally synthesized it had been looking for a drug that could be used in surgery to slow the pulse, heart rate, and other bodily functions. When marketed in the USA, in what has been suggested as 'an at times almost frantic search for therapeutic applications with which (a) to convince the Federal Drug Administration to allow marketing of the drug; and (b) to persuade American physicians to prescribe it',[19] it was considered as a general sedative, a treatment for itching, or control for nausea and vomiting. But it was in its promotion for use with psychotic patients that it really hit the jackpot. It obviously met a need, because just over a year later an estimated 2 million psychiatric patients in the USA were receiving this major tranquillizer. It has been estimated that 150 million people worldwide are on major tranquillizers.[20]

The usual claims for miraculous results were made, although it is still unknown how these drugs actually work. It is a widely accepted part of the official history of psychiatry that the introduction of the major tranquillizers brought about a decline in the population of psychiatric hospitals by enabling many chronic patients to be discharged, and others to stay out of hospital for long periods between admission. Certainly the two events occurred at about the same time, but Scull and others have pointed out that both in the USA and in Britain numbers had begun to fall *before* the new drugs appeared on the market.[21] In Britain, the Open Door Movement had led to the unlocking of wards and the establishing of day hospitals and of therapeutic communities, where staff and patients worked together to break down the roles and rules of the old institutional way of life. Breaking down hierarchies of authority, encouraging emotional expression, making decisions by consensus, and seeing the patients themselves as important sources of help and healing, were the themes of the new settings. This wave of postwar innovation and optimism preceded the new drug treatment in many places; if the major tranquillizers were a factor, they were not the only one, and certainly not the most important one. Recently, reports of one of their most distressing and often irreversible side-effects, tardive dyskinesia, have started to receive wider publicity.

The first anti-depressants to be introduced were the MAOIs. They were discovered accidentally when certain drugs used in the treatment of tuberculosis were found to have a mood-elevating effect. Following a favourable report on their effect on chronically withdrawn patients in 1958 there was a flood of studies and trials (over 1,300 in three years) and widespread enthusiasm about their use. This has now lessened considerably, and the tricyclic group is the usual first choice instead. The tricyclics were discovered accidentally during trials to develop new major tranquillizers, to which they are chemically very similar. The new 'second generation' anti-depressants have been heavily promoted as different and improved versions, although there is little evidence that they are superior to the originals. About 75 million prescriptions for anti-depressants are written annually in Great Britain.[22]

Lithium salts were once used for a variety of ailments, especially gout, but lithium was first suggested as a remedy for the over-excitement of manic patients in 1949 by a doctor who was investigating the toxic effects of injecting uric acid into guinea pigs.[23] In order to carry out this experiment, he first of all had to make the uric acid soluble by adding lithium salts. The result was that the animals became 'extremely lethargic and unresponsive'. Although, as he himself commented rather apologetically, 'it may seem a long distance from lethargy in guinea-pigs to the excitement of psychotics', this did not prevent him from administering lithium to a series of manic patients, and miraculous improvements were claimed. By the 1960s the new treatment was widely used in Europe, although it was slower to catch on in America. One writer has suggested that this 'was due to a lack of enthusiasm on the part of the pharmaceutical companies. Lithium carbonate is such a simple substance that it cannot be patented. . . . The profit margin for manufacturers is therefore a good deal lower than with other products.'[24] One solution to this problem has been to sell lithium in a special slow-release form.

In the 1960s, the first minor tranquillizers appeared on the market. One such tranquillizer was initially promoted as a cure for alcoholism,[25] although it is now known that the two substances are very dangerous in combination and can lead to a dual addiction. The emphasis shifted, via what has been described as 'the slickest and most effective marketing campaign in the history of pharmaceuticals',[26] to selling minor tranquillizers as a simple, non-addictive remedy for anxiety, panic, and other vague and hard-to-define complaints that pose such a problem to GPs and psychiatrists. Promoted in this way the minor tranquillizers (like the major tranquillizers before them) seemed to promise a desperately needed solution to a hitherto enormous and time-consuming problem. Many hard-pressed doctors prescribed them after interviews of less than ten minutes, often without telling patients what they were or warning them about side-effects, and patients could order repeat prescriptions from receptionists for years on end.

The first hints of trouble started to emerge in the late 1970s, when researchers began to uncover some of the less beneficial effects of these drugs. However there was little public or professional awareness of the true scale of the problem until a *That's Life!* TV programme of June 1983 reported the stories of three people who had become dependent on tranquillizers, precipitating jammed switchboards and over 3,000 letters from people recounting similar experiences.[27]

The new treatments paved the way for the next important development from the 1960s onwards: the move from the old Victorian asylums to small psychiatric units attached to district general hospitals. The impetus came partly from the increasing amount of evidence that the asylums were actually creating, rather than curing, the problems that their patients demonstrated. It was 'beyond question that much of the aggressive, disturbed, suicidal, and regressive behaviour of the mentally ill is not necessarily or inherently a part of the illness as such, but is very largely an artificial by-product of the way of life imposed on them'.[28] Since Enoch Powell's impassioned 1961 speech against the 'isolated, majestic, imperious . . . and daunting'[29] asylums, there has been a policy of reducing hospital beds and eventually closing down the old asylums altogether.

At first sight the creation of new units in district general hospitals seems to be a very positive step. Patients and their visitors no longer need to travel miles to vast, grim buildings out in the country, but can instead call in at the new units for outpatient treatment or stay a few days as an in-patient, in the same way as they come up to the general side of the hospital for X-rays or operations. But although these units do have some advantages, they can also be seen as a further victory in the medical profession's campaign to establish psychiatry as just another branch of medicine, to be assimilated with its new drug treatments into the traditional medical world of wards, beds, nurses, and medicines. (Most of the examples in this book are

185

taken from one such unit.) The objections were summarized in a World Health Organization report in 1953:

> In much modern writing on the subject it is taken as axiomatic that psychiatric wards in general hospitals are the most desirable form of provision for psychiatric medical care . . . but, as the committee has emphasized, the psychiatric hospital does not do its job best by imitating the general hospital. Too often the psychiatric wards of a general hospital are forced by the expectations of the hospital authorities to conform to a pattern which is harmful to their purpose. Patients are expected to be in bed and nurses are expected to be engaged in activities which resemble general nursing. The satisfactions of neurological diagnosis are enhanced by the prestige in the general hospital of clear-cut physical pathology, to the detriment of interest in the average psychiatric patient whose case does not exhibit such features . . . the more the psychiatric hospital imitates the general hospital . . . the less successful it will be in creating the atmosphere it needs.'[30]

COMMUNITY CARE

Psychiatry is at present in the middle of the move to what has been designated 'community care'.

The basic idea is that psychiatric services will be based as far as is possible in local facilities such as GP surgeries, clinics, and newly set up Community Mental Health Centres, rather than operating entirely from hospitals. It is hoped that this will reduce the stigma of having to attend a psychiatric hospital, and help the psychiatric service to build closer links with voluntary organizations, Social Services, and local resources. Distressed people will be offered a wider range of options and helped to keep in touch with family, neighbours, and other sources of support. Although a few people will still need to be admitted to hospital, the hope is that additional community support will help them to function outside the hospital most of the time, and the build-up of a chronic, institutionalized hospital population will be avoided. The old asylums are all scheduled for closure, and even patients who have been there for many years are to be rehabilitated back into the outside world. Some areas are considering supplementing or even replacing hospitals with small local crisis units where people can have a temporary break from difficult personal circumstances.

All this sounds very commendable, but whether or not it will turn out to be an improvement in reality is still unclear. The community care movement gains its force from the fact that it appeals both to would-be reformers and to government economists. Reformers hope that the psychiatrists' monopoly will at last be broken, and that Community Mental Health Teams will be made up of a mixture of professionals working together as equals, perhaps headed by a social worker, psychologist, or nurse rather than a doctor. They see community care as a chance to develop a more social and psychotherapeutic approach away from the medical setting of a hospital. However, they are suspicious of governmental enthusiasm for this apparently liberal policy. There is a widespread suspicion that the main appeal of community care is the opportunity it provides for cutting costs under the guise of humanitarian reform. Hospitals are being closed down without enough hostels, day centres, group homes, and so on to replace them. When community care was introduced in America, thousands of psychiatric patients were simply turned out onto the streets; it has been estimated that there are 25,000 homeless mentally ill people in New York alone.[31] There is a danger that CMHCs will end up dealing with the less acute, neurotic end of the spectrum, while the more difficult cases get just as raw a deal as before. Many of Britain's patients will end up being exploited by private landlords, or in doss-houses or sleeping rough, or creating tremendous strain on relatives (usually women) who are forced to take them in, unless enough money is made available to provide alternatives.

Not surprisingly, many of the traditional medical model psychiatrists who make up the majority of the profession are strongly opposed to the philosophy of community care. Although there are genuine reasons for concern, their main anxieties may stem from the fact that they will not necessarily retain their positions as the most important and powerful members of the team, and nor do most of them possess the skills in counselling/psychotherapy which would enable them to carve out a new role for themselves. Other members of staff may also be strongly identified with the traditional system. Especially in the old asylums nurses, for example, can be just as institutionalized as their patients, and find it equally if not more difficult to change.

The crucial question for community care is whether it will be able to live up to its promise of moving away from traditional medical model-style psychiatry. If not, then it will not have been a change for the better. Being diagnosed and medicated in your local clinic is not a great improvement on being diagnosed and medicated in a psychiatric hospital. In fact, extending medical model psychiatry into the community rather than, as at present, having it confined to hospitals, could be seen as a step backwards. For example, there is Project Help, New York's answer to the plight of the homeless mentally distressed, who are rounded up off the streets by psychiatrists or the police and forcibly taken to psychiatric hospital for drug treatment. In Britain, the Royal College of Psychiatrists is campaigning for the introduction of community treatment orders, colloquially known as the 'long leash', under which certain patients would be compelled to take medication even after they have left hospital. This is seen by many as an attempt to extend the power of medical model psychiatrists further into the community. On the other hand, community care could be the start of a very long overdue move towards a whole person, whole system understanding of people in mental distress. What seems to be happening at present is that places which had already started to move away from medical model psychiatry have taken this several steps forward by setting up excellent community-based services, democratically run by skilled and enthusiastic teams; while the more traditional places that make up the majority have either not made any moves at all, or are simply delivering the same old-style service under a different name and in a slightly different setting. The eventual outcome of the community care movements remains to be seen.

The alternative history of psychiatry highlights some remarkable parallels between the nineteenth-century issues, as described by Scull and others, and present-day ones. Now, as then, psychiatry is devoted to proving that mental distress has a physical origin, although there has been no sequel to the discovery that syphilis causes general paralysis of the insane; now, as then, this has increased rather than diminished the search for effective physical treatments to back up the psychiatrists' claims, although explanations of how they work are as speculative as ever and the number of cures (in 1982, out of 155,086 admissions, 133,475 or 85 per cent involved people who had been in at least once before)[32] remains distressingly low; now, as then, there is no shortage of jargon and obscure lists of diagnoses to give the whole field of psychiatry an air of authority and special expertise. Community care is the most serious threat to medical model psychiatry since the era of moral treatment, and many psychiatrists are reacting to it, as they have reacted to other non-medical approaches like psychotherapy, in exactly the same way. 'Of course it has some valuable aspects . . . important part of any good service . . . long been aware of need to incorporate such factors', etc. etc., but the only profession that is properly qualified to combine all the relevant areas of knowledge and control the whole enterprise is the medical one.

As we saw with moral treatment in the nineteenth century, this reduces a whole philosophy of care to a mere set of extra skills possessed by the medical profession, while the medical model remains the basic approach. It remains to be seen whether this manoeuvre will strangle community care as it did moral treatment (which, it can be shown, produced the highest rate of cures that psychiatry has achieved before or since).[33] Meanwhile modern psychiatry's main claims to success are either inaccurate (e.g. that the major tranquillizers enabled chronic patients to be discharged); or consist of belated recognition of the harmfulness of some of its earlier treatments:

British psychiatry . . . has earned itself a distinguished record for its exploration of the aetiological role of social factors in psychiatric illness. The work of researchers in Britain showed that many of the psychiatrical and behavioural features exhibited by chronic mental hospital inmates owed more to the manner whereby such patients were treated than to the actual illness . . .[34]

or represent a return to the ideals of moral treatment while staying just within the medical model (e.g. Leff's work, which shows, not very surprisingly, that patients diagnosed as schizophrenic do better in a supportive atmosphere that is not too hostile or critical).

The drug revolution of the 1950s and 1960s seemed to provide the validation, awaited since the early nineteenth century, of psychiatrists' claims to have special knowledge and expertise in the treatment of the mentally distressed. It certainly convinced many people — see Sir Keith Joseph's speech earlier in the chapter.

But are the current physical treatments for psychiatric patients a genuine advance on the previous ones? To what extent, for example, can the seventy-plus minor tranquillizers and the equal number of major tranquillizers currently on the market be said to be an improvement on the thirty-four emetics and fifty purgatives of the nineteenth century? Is the shock of ten ECTs essentially different from the shock of ten pails of icy water? Or are these just the latest versions of moves in the same old game? These questions will be considered in the next chapter.

Physical treatments and the role
of the drug industry

It is impossible to evaluate the true impact of the new drug treatments of the 1950s and 60s without taking a close look at the role of the pharmaceutical (drug) industry in psychiatry.

Pharmaceutical companies are among the most powerful and profitable on earth. In fact they have been ranked first or second most profitable industries in the world in most years since 1955.[1] 'The multinationals have financial strength that in many cases exceeds that of many governments . . . Each of the ten largest multinationals earns annual revenues greater than the gross national products of two-thirds of the countries in the world.'[2] It has been estimated that the marker for one company is about 100 million dollars a year from these drugs in America alone,[3] while in Britain, where minor tranquillizers are by far the most commonly prescribed drugs, enough of them were distributed in 1981 to allow for thirty tablets for every man, woman, and child in the country.[4] Diazepam is reported to be the most widely prescribed drug in the world.[5] The major tranquillizers are a similar success story for the drug industry; an estimated 150 million people take them worldwide.[6] Drug companies spend around £5,000 a year on every GP in Britain or £150 million a year in total[7] to promote their products and the annual NHS drugs bill is around £2,000 million.

Obviously, where such enormous sums of money are involved, drug companies have a very strong vested interest in selling the chemical solution to mental distress. Of course, this does not necessarily mean that their products are of no value. However, it does mean that where there is a conflict between public service and making money and between giving accurate information and making sales, it is not always the worthier motive that carries the day.

The particular structure of the pharmaceutical industry means that huge profits are virtually guaranteed, regardless of economic recessions and competitive market forces. The industry is half way to being a monopoly: the top thirty drug companies in the world control more than 60 per cent of the market.[8] Moreover there is strong evidence of unofficial agreements between the various companies to fix their prices at very similar levels, since they would all lose out if there was a price-cutting war.[9] Instead, companies tend to specialize in different fields, so that one will make antibiotics while another produces tranquillizers or contraceptives. Again, since the doctors who prescribe drugs are not picking up the bill for them, there is no need for them to be price-conscious in their choices. Yet another factor that limits competition and thus keeps prices high is the system of giving patents. A company which discovers a new drug is, in many countries, granted a patent for a certain length of time (twenty years in Britain) during which it alone can manufacture and sell its new product. When the patent expires, any company can make and sell the drug under its generic name. But an effective campaign will ensure that the brand name remains in doctors' minds, so that even when the patent runs out doctors will automatically continue to prescribe the brand version. Eight years after one company's patent on its product expired, it still held 75 per cent of the market for it, even though its brand name version cost significantly more than the generic version.[10] Another result is that other drug companies pour enormous proportions of their research money (one estimate is 75 per cent)[11] into producing what are known as 'me-too' drugs — products that are just different enough from the patented one to earn their own patent. Although heavily promoted as new, exciting, and different, such products are virtually indistinguishable in practice from the original one, and merely add to the confusing choice of drugs facing the doctor (around 6,500 in Britain). The official justification of the patenting system is that it allows companies time to recoup the enormous costs of research (for each product that reaches the market, about 5,000 compounds will have been discarded along the way).[12] However, the overall effect, again, is to limit competition to keep prices high. The drug companies have a number of ways of maintaining this happy (for them) state of affairs, some less admirable than others. Their front line consists of the drug company sales people or 'drug reps' (one for every seven GPs in Britain) who are trained to promote their company's products on their regular visits to surgeries and hospitals. Other methods can be summarized under three main headings.

ADVERTISING

Drug companies spend vast sums of money on adverts in medical journals and on the free drug-firm literature that GPs receive through the post, estimated by one researcher at thirty-five journals and fifty adverts for each doctor every month. The range of problems for which a chemical solution has been proposed is enormous: one product was initially recommended for alcoholism, anxiety, tense muscles, and cardiovascular problems,[13] and also for tricky cases like the 'always weary', 'psychic support for the tense insomniac', and even to create 'a less demanding and complaining patient'. Another was said to be of use for, among other things, the college student whose 'newly stimulated intellectual curiosity may make her more sensitive to and apprehensive about unstable national and world conditions'.[14] Faced with a cure looking for a disease, the drug industry has been ingenious in defining new illnesses and hence new applications for its products. The minor tranquillizers in particular 'have been promoted as solutions to almost every state which falls short of total serenity'.[15]

Drug adverts are notorious for presenting women in a stereotyped and unflattering way. After a lengthy search through medical journals, two investigators could only find two advertisements that depicted a woman as the doctor or therapist. More typical were those such as the one which

> portrays the tear-streaked face of an attractive young blonde woman who is said to be suffering from 'copelessness'. Medication, it is suggested, will help her pull herself together and apply herself to needed tasks. These advertisements strongly suggest that inability to function in a traditional female role, inability to cope with being a woman and with women's tasks, need to be treated with medication.[16]

Similarly, 'Mrs Hunter', another young blonde and a

housewife and mother — she complains of feeling unable to cope, being constantly irritable and shouting at the children', receives the diagnosis 'depression with presenting anxiety symptoms' and the instant solution — an anti-depressant.

In addition, advertisements may make misleading references to research papers, while studies that give less favourable results are omitted or glossed over.

INFILTRATION

This term refers to the many subtle and not-so-subtle strategies by which drug companies ensure that their products form the background to just about every medical activity. Gifts stamped with the company and product name — pens, blotters, clocks, paperweights, calendars, notepads, textbooks, pencil cases, name stamps, files, paperclip holders, leaflet displays, and so on — are given out to medical students and fill the GP's office. Free samples are handed out by the drug reps, while doctors have been offered watches, microwaves, televisions, and all sorts of consumer durables as a reward for prescribing certain products. Drug companies lend or give equipment to surgeries and hospitals. They provide films and publications for medical training. Senior doctors and their spouses may be funded to fly to conferences in exotic places with trips, amenities, and entertainment laid on — and, of course, the relevant company's products prominently displayed. 'Drug lunches', at which food far superior to that of the average hospital canteen is served after a film about the wonders of some new pill, are a regular feature of hospital life. Drug companies underwrite the cost of meetings, seminars, and conferences in return for the opportunity to put their name on the programme and send their drug reps to set up stalls at the event. They make contributions to party political funds.[17] Even if doctors remain fairly cynical about particular claims and tactics, the overall effect is to create a culture where the solution to a patient's problems is assumed to be a chemical one.

It is alarming to realize how crucially the drug companies are involved even in apparently more objective information about their products and medical issues in general. Medical journals rely on funds from drug advertisements and may not be able to afford to offend the industry. (One researcher had an article on the image of women in these advertisements rejected by twenty different journals.)[18] Drug companies fund foreign fellowships and underwrite the cost of television programmes. Doctors may be offered money for every patient they treat with a certain drug in a 'research trial' which has the underlying aim of getting patients switched to the new product. More crucially, the fact that the drug industry funds medical research in universities, hospitals, and medical schools means that investigations into non-drug and non-medical approaches are much harder to fund, and are correspondingly less likely to get off the ground. Members of government drug regulatory bodies may also be, or have been, in the pay of the drug industry at other times in their lives. One of the main international doctors' pocketbooks on drugs (Monthly Index of Medical Specialties, or MIMS) relies on information supplied by the companies themselves. It does not, contrary to popular belief, generally list adverse effects, and editions for Third World countries where regulations are less strict may include products that are banned elsewhere.[19]

In some countries the companies themselves supply the pharmacology teachers for the medical schools. This has particularly tragic implications for the Third World; for example, 400 million dollars worth of anti-diarrhoeal drugs are prescribed globally, often to parents who can barely afford to buy them, and yet most of the 5 million children who die of diarrhoea every year could be saved by a simple and cheap mixture of water, sugar, and salt.[20] But since there is no profit in this for the drug companies, there is no incentive to teach it to medical students.

This category shades over into the next one:

CORRUPTION

Dr John Braithwaite, who has investigated this subject in depth, found that 'corporate crime is a bigger problem in the pharmaceutical industry than any other'. To start with,

My own research found evidence of substantial bribery by 19 of the 20 largest American pharmaceutical companies. There is evidence of bribes being paid to every type of government official who could conceivably affect the interests of pharmaceutical companies: bribes to cabinet ministers to get drugs approved for marketing; bribes to social security bureaucrats who fix prices for subsidized drugs; to health inspectors who check pharmaceutical manufacturing plants; to customs officials, hospital administrators, tax assessors, political parties, and others.

Safety testing procedures provided further examples of fraud:

Rats die in trials on new drugs and are replaced with live animals; rats which develop tumours are replaced with healthy rats; doctors who are being paid 1,000 dollars a patient to test a new product pour the pills down the toilet, making up the results in a way which tells the company what it wants to hear.[21]

Other scandals abound. Drugs that have been banned in the West can be 'dumped' in the Third World by strategies such as changing the name, altering the formula slightly, setting up a factory in a country with less strict regulations, and so on.[22] Drugs which are regarded as too high-risk for testing in the West can be tried out in the Third World instead.[23] Latin American health ministers are 'almost invariably rich with wealth which comes largely from the international pharmaceutical industry'.[24] The list goes on. Moreover, the very power which enables the companies to act in this way makes it hard, if not impossible, to bring them to account. When the Daily Mirror serialized a book called *Health Shock* which was critical of the drug industry, 'constant phone calls at home, threatening cables, and telexes sent to the Mirror's chief lawyer and editor put immense pressure on the newspaper'.[25] In the thalidomide disaster the company never admitted liability, nor was a court judgment ever passed on it; the trial dragged on for two and a half years and the company then settled out of court. Dr Braithwaite writes, 'To my knowledge at least, the thalidomide disaster led to not one successful prosecution nor one successful private law suit in a court of law anywhere in the world'.[26]

At the same time, Braithwaite pointed out that many, indeed most, drug industry executives and employees are honest, idealistic, and highly committed to responsible business conduct. Fraud flourishes in this situation partly because of the complexity of the organization — most people will have no knowledge of or contact with corrupt conduct — and partly because employees are only involved in doing their own small piece of the work to the best of their ability.

Consider, for example, the quality control manager who is exacting in ensuring that no drug leaves the plant which is impure or outside specifications. It might be that the drug itself causes more harm than good because of side-effects or abuse; but the quality control manager does the job of ensuring that at least it is not adulterated.[27]

So, 'the difference between socially responsible and corrupt companies is that in the former, ethical questions are everyone's business'.[28]

Although all governments have tried to reduce the NHS drugs bill and have had some form of drug price control, the threat of combined opposition from the medical profession (who want to preserve their clinical freedom to prescribe what they think best) and from the drug industry has been a serious impediment. One recommendation made by the Informal Working Group on Effective Prescribing, known as the Greenfield Report, in 1982, was that pharmacists should automatically dispense the cheaper generic version of any drug unless the doctor specifically indicated a preference for the brand version.[29] This was never implemented. Although this policy (generic substitution) has been practised in British hospital pharmacies for some time, the drug industry successfully argued that if it was introduced at a wider level there would be 'far-reaching and damaging effects on the welfare of patients, the national economy and even on the practice of medicine'.[30] However, governments find that there are compensations to this awkward dilemma. The increasing power of the drug industry means that it contributes a net £600 million a year to the balance of trade by exporting its products[31] — far more than could be saved on the drugs bill. The Government, the medical profession, and the drug industry each benefit from the co-operation of the other. 'British government policy is that medicines should help people *and* the national economy to get better and stay well: too bad if these objectives conflict'.[32]

New physical treatments in psychiatry all tend to go through predictable cycles of opinion. The initial discovery is accidental: 'A clinician has used a drug for the treatment of psychiatric patients, usually on quite false theoretical grounds, and found clinical effects that he had never predicted'.[33] The treatment is initially greeted with cries of wonder and delight, and a flood of reports glowingly describe its safe and miraculous action in all sorts of previously problematic conditions. One of the first minor tranquillizers to be developed was said at various times to give symptomatic relief in alcoholism, allergies, angina pectoris, appendicitis, asthma, behavioural disorders in children, depression, skin problems, glaucoma, hypertension, intractable pain, childbirth, menopause, motion sickness, petit mal epilepsy, stuttering, typhoid fever, and half a dozen other ailments.[34] And here is an American psychiatrist extolling the effects of the new major tranquillizers on institutional life:

> A transformation has occurred in mental hospitals in the past two decades that defies description. Visit one today. You will be impressed by the serenity you observe and feel. Flowers, curtains, paintings, music, fresh air, comfortable tidy lounges make a pleasant environment for clean, tranquil patients being offered a myriad of therapies.[35]

Here is another psychiatrist extolling lithium:

> Manic depression, this spectacular disease, now has an equally spectacular cure. Lithium is the first drug in the history of psychiatry to so radically and specifically control a major mind disorder. . . . It is truly spectacular to watch this simple, naturally occurring salt . . . return a person in one to three weeks from the terrible throes of mood-swing to normalcy.[36]

And again, a psychiatrist recommending ECT for, among other things, heroin withdrawal, colitis, psoriasis, schizophrenia, and the pain associated with back ailments and cancer: 'Surely shock treatment represents one of those medical miracles that the *Reader's Digest* likes to write about.'[37]

(Similar claims were made in 1898 for a new drug that was safe, non-addictive, effective in controlling pain and in infant respiratory ailments and a cure for morphine addiction. It performed so heroically that it was named heroin.)[38]

After a while it becomes clear that the new treatment is neither as effective nor as widely applicable as was first claimed, but it is still viewed as very useful in a more limited range of situations and becomes one of the standard tools of psychiatry.

Finally, evidence begins to mount that the treatment is either useless, of very limited use, or even positively harmful. (One recent example of this is insulin coma therapy. Barbiturates were once widely prescribed where minor tranquillizers would be used now and amphetamines were recommended for as many different disorders as the minor tranquillizers in the early days of their use, but especially for depression before the days of anti-depressants. It is now recognized that both these classes of drugs are highly addictive and very dangerous in overdose and they are Controlled Drugs under the Misuse of Drugs Act of 1971). The treatment is abandoned, and the whole cycle starts again with something else.

The current favourite physical treatments in psychiatry can be seen as occupying various positions in this cycle. The minor tranquillizers, although still used, have taken a severe knocking as their very serious drawbacks (withdrawal symptoms and the like) have become apparent. ECT and the major tranquillizers are somewhere in the middle stage of the cycle; although their limitations are acknowledged, at least to some extent, they are still widely and routinely used. However, sources other than the official ones of psychiatry textbooks and medical journals (which, as we have seen, may not always be as impartial as one would wish) provide some disquieting evidence about their effects. The major tranquillizers are, in my opinion, the current most likely candidates to enter the final stage of the cycle.

It maybe useful to consider each of these treatments in more detail.

MINOR TRANQUILLIZERS

There is now widespread public and professional awareness of the potential dangers of these drugs and many GPs and psychiatrists have altered their prescribing habits accordingly. Some people in the *That's Life!* survey on tranquillizers had found them very useful for short periods of time or during particular crises. However, a MORI poll indicated that one-third of the one in four British adults who have taken a tranquillizer at some time in their lives had been on them for more than four months (the time beyond which they are ineffective).[39] Some had been taking them for 10 or 20 years. The majority of these people were women (as were the users of barbiturates and amphetamines).

The demand for some kind of pill to take away emotional distress often comes from patients, although it is an equally welcome solution to many doctors who, misinformed by the drug companies, handed out tranquillizers with the assurance that they were not addictive. The pills sometimes seemed to help for a while until other symptoms developed. Not realizing that these symptoms were in fact *caused* by the drugs, the natural assumption to make was that the illness was getting worse.

The solution suggested by the equally ignorant doctors was often to increase the dosage, and the effects on the patient and her or his family life continued: 'I'm afraid I feel that those years were wasted. I floated through everything. I missed a lot of my children's upbringing, I've forgotten so much. Looking back it was like being in a cocoon.'[41] 'I didn't feel I was fit to take my children out alone as I had panic attacks, sweating, and peculiar breathing. Very antisocial, completely different person in fact. Couldn't concentrate on conversations with people.'[42]

Coming off the pills often led to even worse problems, and again since the tablets were supposed to be non-addictive, these were mistaken for a return of the original problem. Not everyone suffers withdrawal symptoms. For those who do, though, cutting down can be a nightmare; indeed, a leading psychiatrist has said that it is much worse coming off a particular minor tranquillizer than heroin.[43] Experiences such as this bear him out:

> I would feel myself becoming very weak and it even affected my voice. I would shake and my heart would beat so fast that sleep was impossible. I felt like my whole insides were shaking and some mornings I had to be sick I felt so ill, for months. I laid about feeling so ill. . . . If I did fall asleep I would wake up, because my whole body kept jerking. I felt so ill that all I did was cry, it really was hell. I hardly ate anything for months. . . . My skin turned a funny colour; to me it looked yellow. . . . My eyes hurt all the time and have sunk through being so ill.[44]

Minor tranquillizers may have other consequences too. One study found that people taking them were five times more likely to have accidents at work, in the home, or on the roads. Use of these drugs has been linked with birth defects such as cleft palates. In elderly people, the side effects can be confused with senility.[45]

The most recent recommendation of the Committee on the Safety of Medicine is that minor tranquillizers should be used for a maximum of four weeks and only for a limited range of problems, for example, for anxiety or insomnia that is 'severe, disabling and subjecting the individual to extreme stress', and not for mild anxiety or phobic or obsessional states. The Committee warns that 'withdrawal symptoms can occur with benzodiazepines following therapeutic doses given for *short* period of time.'[46] And now 150 lawyers, representing more than 1,000 tranquillizer victims, are planning to take legal action based on 'the mass of evidence showing that the medical profession and the drug companies knew many years ago that there were major problems with these drugs, but did not act in their patients' interest to limit the damage they were likely to cause.'[47]

NHS facilities for coming off tranquillizers do exist but they are few and far between. Voluntary bodies like Tranx and Release have done much to fill the gap.

MAJOR TRANQUILLIZERS

The major tranquillizers are seen as psychiatry's most effective treatment for schizophrenia. The antipsychotic drugs have emerged as a routine, almost automatic, remedy in psychosis and relatively little effort has been made in psychiatry to use these medicines selectively. 'One might search for a long time to find a diagnosed schizophrenic who has never been treated with a neuroleptic drug.'[46] They are also sometimes recommended to control mania (when a person becomes restless, supercharged with energy, and very 'high'), and to relieve severe anxiety.

The major tranquillizers do not cure schizophrenia or anything else, but they do suppress the more distressing symptoms of the acute stages of a breakdown, and taken over a longer period of time they enable many people to lead a reasonably normal life outside hospital, and, it is argued, help prevent relapse. Clearly they have their uses, but in making an overall assessment of their value the questions that need to be asked are first, at what price these benefits are bought, second, to how many people this applies, and third, how they are actually used in day-to-day practice.

The major tranquillizers are not pleasant drugs to take, although of course they may be preferable to the alternatives (hearing voices and so on). The problem of compliance (getting reluctant patients to carry on with their medication) has been partly solved by administering them in the form of slow-release injections. Restlessness is one side effect ('It may not mean much to you but I feel all squishy inside in the morning. Kind of jittery-like. I just don't feel comfortable . . . I used to work in an office but I can't do that any more. I just can't sit all day'),[49] as is general sedation ('I was far more alive when I was hearing voices and more normal to myself, more an extension of my normal self . . . since I've been on medication it's debilitating to say the least').[50] Other possible side effects are blurred vision, weight-gain, impotence, apathy, dry mouth, and sensitivity of the skin to sunlight. In addition there are two potential results, pseudo-Parkinsonism and tardive dyskinesia, which are more serious.

Pseudo-Parkinsonism

Some people taking major tranquillizers, especially if they are on a high dosage, experience the very unpleasant symptoms of Parkinson's disease, which include a mask-like face, an open and dribbling mouth, shaky hands, and shuffling walk. More medication (anti-cholinergic drugs) may be prescribed to control these symptoms. However, this has two disadvantages: one, that these drugs themselves have side effects like constipation, dizziness, and blurred vision, and two, that they may increase the risk of developing the even more serious condition, tardive dyskinesia.

Tardive dyskinesia

Tardive dyskinesia is characterized by uncontrollable movements of the lip, tongue, and face, fidgeting hands, tapping feet, rocking backwards and forwards, grunting, and other bizarre involuntary mannerisms. If the major tranquillizers are stopped as soon as the first signs are detected these movements generally disappear. Often, though, the symptoms of tardive dyskinesia only emerge when a patient cuts down on or stops his or her medication — sometimes weeks or months later. Again, the movements may gradually fade, but some people are left with a permanent, irreversible disability for which the only 'treatment' is to go back on the major tranquillizers again. The trap in doing this is that although the symptoms of tardive dyskinesia will once more be masked, in the long term the drugs will increase the neurological damage that led to the problem in the first place.

In accordance with the cycles of opinion that we have already discussed, the risks attached to these new wonder-drugs were hardly mentioned for many years — indeed the major tranquillizers were described as 'among the safest drugs available in medicine'.[51] Some writers have argued that there has been a semi-deliberate cover-up of the facts about tardive dyskinesia by the professionals leading to an 'almost total denial of the phenomenon in the 1950s and early 1960s'.[50] The preface to the first book on the subject (published in 1980, by which time the drugs had been on the market for over twenty-five years) noted that the literature on tardive dyskinesia contained

> hardly an impressive number of reports and certainly small by comparison to the prolific output of psycho-pharmacologists in other areas. . . . The majority of psychiatrists either ignored the existence of the problem or made futile efforts to prove that these motor abnormalities were clinically insignificant or unrelated to drug therapy.[51]

Currently there is much more public and professional awareness of the issue, although far less than in America where patients who developed tardive dyskinesia have successfully sued psychiatrists for not informing them about the risks. However it is still very hard to get accurate figures on how many of the people who take major tranquillizers will develop tardive dyskinesia; on one estimate, 10 to 20 per cent of patients in psychiatric hospitals and 40 per cent of the elderly who have been on long-term drug therapy are at risk.[54] One drug company has put the risk at only 3 to 6 per cent, which would still mean that 5 to 10 million people worldwide have tardive dyskinesia.[55] Others have argued that this is a serious underestimate and that the true figure for irreversible tardive dyskinesia is nearer 21 million, or about 1 to 2 million cases a year,[56] making it 'among the worst medically-induced disasters in history'.[57]

Three further consequences of using major tranquillizers, seldom addressed in the literature, deserve a mention. The first is the stigma that results from the changes in appearance and behaviour described above. Patients affected in this way look odd and crazy, with their blank faces, grimaces, and shuffling walk. As well as being distressing to them, their relatives, and other patients, this is a serious hindrance to being accepted back into everyday life. Although any member of the public who took a stroll round a psychiatric hospital might conclude that these bizarre mannerisms, together with the pervasive apathy and list-lessness of the patients, were the result of mental illness, in fact they are caused by the treatment. The second damaging conse-quence is that this apathy (the inevitable result of taking such powerful sedatives) undermines the ability of patients to take advantage of social programmes and work training, especially since there is evidence that the major tranquillizers impair learning ability.[58] The third and very important hazard is that withdrawal from major tranquillizers may cause psychiatric symptoms to rebound to a higher level than they would other-wise have reached — in other words, that in some circumstances the treatment may actually cause the problem for which it purports to be the cure. Almost universally unaware of this possibility, psychiatrists regard sudden relapses when major tranquillizers are reduced or stopped as a sure indication that the drugs are playing an essential role in keeping the condition under control, and prescribing is started up again. Failure to take this phenomenon (known as tardive psychosis) into account means that many research studies on drug withdrawal give a misleading impression of the efficacy of these drugs. Again, as with tardive dyskinesia, a vicious circle is set up. Continuing the drugs may mask the psychiatric symptoms again, but only at the expense of worsening the underlying problem, so that patients 'must remain on neuroleptics for the rest of their life regardless of the natural course of the illness'.[59]

The possible explanation for tardive psychosis is complex and has been well summarized by Warner.[60] Briefly, he starts from the current hypothesis that in people diagnosed as schizophrenic there is overactivity in some of the nerve pathways which use a certain chemical, dopamine, to transmit messages from one cell to another. (This, if true, is very unlikely to be a simple and direct causal factor, if it is one at all — see Chapter 4.) The chemical messages are picked up by specific receptors in the nerve cells, and it is thought that major tranquillizers work by blocking these receptors and thus reducing the level of activity in the nerve pathways. There is some evidence that the original overactivity is not caused by an excessive amount of dopamine but by excessive sensitivity on the part of the receptors. When the receptors are blocked by drugs, the body may compensate by making them even more sensitive to dopamine. This does not matter as long as the drugs continue to have their blocking effect, but if they are stopped, the artificial sensitivity that they have created can lead to very serious consequences: to tardive psychosis if the sensitivity occurs in one set of nerve pathways, and/or to tardive dyskinesia if it occurs in another set. In other words, although the short-term effects of major tranquillizers may be beneficial, 'the long-term effect . . . *may be a worsening of the basic neurochemical defect in schizophrenia'*.

Warner believes that for patients with a poor prognosis, the benefits of the major tranquillizers may still outweigh the disadvantages. However, he argues that for the 50 per cent or so of patients whose prognosis is good (i.e. their breakdown came on suddenly and after an identifiable stress, or later on in life, and they were previously functioning well), 'drug withdrawal may worsen the course of an otherwise benign condition and drug maintenance therapy may increase the risk of psychosis, cause side-effects, or, at best, prove worthless'.[61] In support of this statement he quotes various studies comparing drug and non-drug treatment in patients with good and with poor prognosis, which demonstrate that patients with good prognosis actually do worse (in terms of symptoms and readmission to hospital) on major tranquillizers than without them. Conclusions such as, 'Antipsychotic medication is not the treatment of choice, at least for certain patients, if one is interested in long-term clinical improvement' were drawn by the investigators.[62]

A more outspoken critic of psychiatric drugs and of major tranquillizers in particular is American psychiatrist Peter Breggin.[63] He argues that major tranquillizers have no specific effect at all, and that their impact is not only on the dopamine systems but on nearly all other biochemical reactions in the brain as well. In fact, he believes that they achieve their effect by disabling the brain in a manner similar to a lobotomy. Among the evidence he cites in support of his argument is the very high rate of generalized brain disease and dementia in patients with tardive dyskinesia, the frightening implications of which have been played down or ignored by investigators.[64] He also quotes various studies whose disturbing conclusions ('It is also clear that the antipsychotic drugs must continue to be scrutinized for the possibility that their extensive consumption might cause general brain dysfunction'.[65] and so on) have somehow been overlooked in subsequent research and review articles.

In the light of all this evidence, it is a matter of great concern that the major tranquillizers are used so routinely, in such high doses, and often in such dangerous combinations.

> Patients of all ages have told MIND that major tranquillizers are being prescribed in combination with other similar drugs at dosages close to, or higher than, recommended levels. . . . There is *no* medical reason to prescribe several different major tranquillizers at once and doing so may increase the risk of tardive dyskinesia as well as causing patients unnecessary discomfort from a combination of side-effects. It may be correct in unusual circumstances, for example a short-lived emergency, to prescribe a major tranquillizer at a very high dosage. However, long-term use of these drugs at high dosages gives rise to considerable concern.[66]

Even more alarming is the use of major tranquillizers on groups of people for whom they are often clearly inappropriate: the elderly, the mentally handicapped, and prisoners. MIND again:

> Older people are much more likely to experience side-effects from drugs, so major tranquillizers should be prescribed with particular care and sensitivity. . . . There is a worrying number of cases where major tranquillizers are wrongly prescribed, or given at too high a dosage. Between 30 and 60 per cent of mentally handicapped people in hospital are on long-term prescriptions for major tranquillizers. . . . In many cases it seems that major tranquillizers have been prescribed where *no* mental illness has been diagnosed: these powerful drugs are obviously being used as sedatives in order to make mentally handicapped people more manageable. . . . It is a matter for serious concern that many mentally handicapped people will be unable to express their worries or distress about the side-effects of major tranquillizers and it is highly likely that some of the contorted facial expressions and agitated behaviour displayed by mentally handicapped people are a direct result of those drugs. There is also recent evidence to suggest that long-term use of major tranquillizers leads to more disturbed behaviour in mentally handicapped people and seriously affects their ability to learn.[67]

MIND also notes that there are frequent allegations of these drugs being used for purposes of control in prisons, while in psychiatric hospitals 'it often happens that more drugs are prescribed where there is a shortage of nursing staff, or the staff are under pressure.' In such cases the line between treatment and control becomes dangerously blurred.

ECT (ELECTRO-CONVULSIVE THERAPY)

ECT is given in a special room where the patient lies on a bed and is given a general anaesthetic and a muscle relaxant. Padded electrodes are placed on her head and an electric current of about eighty volts is passed through her brain. She will probably wake up confused and with a headache, and will need to rest for about an hour afterwards. Standard length courses of ECT consist of 4 to 12 individual shocks given a few days apart.

The official current view of ECT is that although no one knows exactly how it works, 'there is substantial and incontrovertible evidence that the ECT procedure is an effective treatment in severe depressive illness'.[68] One standard textbook sees it as particularly valuable in depression in middle age, where 'about 80 per cent of the cases respond, the illness is in most instances cut short, suffering is much reduced and management facilitated'. This is obviously a very desirable outcome, especially since according to the same textbook 'there is no evidence that a previously normal brain suffers permanent damage of any consequence from a standard course of ECT', although 'during the treatment course and for a week or two subsequently many patients complain of forgetfulness, particularly over dates, names, and such details'.[69] A British review article came to similar conclusions, and although noting 'the widespread conviction by former patients that their memories have been permanently affected', dismisses these effects as neither serious nor extensive and attributes the complaints to a 'heightened awareness of normal failings. . . . It is well known in other contexts that there is little correlation between subjective complaint and objective impairment where memory is concerned'.[70] Despite what the Royal College of Psychiatrists calls 'poorly informed public comments on the effects and effectiveness of ECT'[71] it is very widely used (about 200,000 treatments a year) although this varies a great deal from place to place, with some hospitals giving it up to seventeen times as much as others.[72] It is sometimes recommended for mania or schizophrenia as well. The early custom of giving regular treatments to prevent relapse, so that individual patients might receive several hundred rounds of ECT, has fortunately been abandoned.

The official account can be balanced by the alternative view provided by investigators such as Peter Breggin, whose book *Electroshock — Its Brain-disabling Effects*[73] analyses the hundreds of medical research papers on the effects of ECT on the brain. His conclusions are not reassuring. In brief, he argues that there is in fact very little evidence that ECT is helpful and a good deal of evidence that it can be very harmful in any quantity, both in the short-term and the long-term. Moreover he believes that ECT achieves its effects in a way that is not at all mysterious — by damaging the brain, often permanently. In other words he sees it, as he sees the major tranquillizers, as a slightly more sophisticated version of lobotomy.

Breggin points out that immediately after ECT the patient suffers from the same acute confusional syndrome that occurs after any trauma to the brain, whether the result of epilepsy, strangulation, suffocation, blows to the head, or lobotomy. She (and it usually is a she, in the ratio 2.27 to 1)[74] is confused and disoriented with impaired judgement and insight and all her intellectual functions disrupted, and may display shallow or inappropriate emotional reactions. She may find herself with a severe headache, nausea, and a feeling of being out of touch with reality. This acute stage wears off over the next hour or two. The more serious effects do not disappear so quickly, if at all, and Breggin presents evidence that although longer courses of treatment produce more severe damage, it can also occur after standard length courses.

The commonest effects are loss of memory for events that took place before the ECT was given (reterograde amnesia), and/or loss of memory for events that occur after the ECT (anterograde amnesia). Memory loss may span all areas of life experience. Thus, patients may be unable to recall educational and professional experiences; films, books and plays; important social events such as birthdays and family gatherings; names and faces of friends and acquaintances; household details such as how to do the chores and where things are kept; familiar locations such as the layout of the local shops or town; what happened to them in hospital; inner thoughts and feelings; and public events such as elections and news stories. Obviously this can be extremely distressing. In one woman's words:

> There are a lot of blanks that have to be pieced together for me. Sometimes when I get very frustrated and angry, I ask my husband or father to tell me different things that I've known since childhood, like my relatives and uncles, and what my children's names were, and where they were and what they did. I always had a very good knowledge of this because I had been the one in the family who kept in communication and kept the family aware of each other's doings. . . . But I cannot go back and feel the feelings I had then. I told my sister one day that I don't remember the things shown in the pictures from my honeymoon, but I can see a happy female in the photographs. The experience is lost. I have the data that somebody gave me, I have the pictures, and therefore I know it did occur. But the actual physical feeling of being there — no, it's gone.[75]

Another woman said,

> Returning to a home and family following shock was a truly bewildering experience. I had entirely forgotten how to accomplish even the simplest tasks. . . . It was like moving into the home of a complete stranger — myself. Many times I have felt like a second wife; I often find traces and marks of the other wife and feel she was then a much better person than I am today.[76]

In addition, Breggin argues that patients may be left with a more general permanent impairment, such as difficulty in understanding what is heard or read, in doing simple sums, in concentrating, in learning new tasks, and in many other areas. In other words, ECT may, in some cases, and particularly in large amounts, result in severe, global, and permanent brain damage.

Some degree of reterograde and anterograde amnesia is an effect widely acknowledged by ECT's advocates, although as we have seen they usually describe it as mild and short-lived. The possibility of more serious memory loss and a more general loss of brain function is hardly mentioned at all, certainly not where standard length courses of ECT are concerned. The situation is complicated by the fact that those patients who are most severely impaired tend to complain the least. Like sufferers from senile dementia, they tend to confabulate — i.e. to cover up the gaps in their memories by faking recollections or by denying difficulties which later show up on neurological and psychological tests. Some conceal their difficulties out of shame or embarrassment, while others have been accused of exaggerating. However, it ought not to come as a surprise that ECT can have such devastating effects. Breggin points out that Cerletti and Bini, the Italian inventors of ECT, had to abandon their early experiments on dogs' brains because of the severity of the resulting brain damage. He also notes that the idea that ECT works by destroying brain tissue was a widely acknowledged and not particularly controversial one in the early days of its use, especially in America where it was a relatively mild intervention compared to some of the other physical treatments that were in vogue (for example, forcing mental patients to breathe nitrogen until they collapsed, or freezing them into a coma by packing them in ice). Research papers and textbooks of the time presented evidence that the ECT patient 'secures his re-adaptation to normal life at the expense of a permanent lowering of functional efficiency. He may, in the language of chess, be sacrificing a piece to win the game'.[77] This was seen (at least by the doctors) as an acceptable compromise, and no reason to limit the very wide and enthusiastic use of the new treatment. However after 1947, when a committee of America's most eminent psychiatrists expressed grave doubts about the abuses of ECT,[78] there was a dramatic change of attitude. From that date, according to Breggin, there was a tendency for reviews and textbooks either to fail to mention research which warned about serious brain damage, or else to misrepresent its conclusions, while evidence quoted in support of the use of ECT was often unsound or misleading. Breggin gives a number of examples from different areas. In the field of animal research the adverse effects that emerged from the original experiments on dogs were played down, with claims that no permanent damage had occured, an assertion that has been repeated by subsequent reviewers. Among a number of animal studies which supported the opposite conclusion was an extensive and widely ignored investigation by Hartelius[79] who found that even on conservative criteria ECT can produce irreversible brain damage. In the field of clinical reports, accounts of patients who have been left with considerable memory problems are not included in reviews. Some researchers claim that ECT does not result in any permanent memory loss,[80] whereas Breggin claims that the papers on which the conclusions are based tend to support the opposite conclusion if anything. He claims the same to be the case for the fields of human autopsy studies and human brainwave and neurological studies. He argues that after a time these conclusions acquire the status of accepted facts and are quoted unquestioningly in reviews and textbooks, while more critical accounts of ECT (and of other psychiatric treatments) only tend to appear when a competing treatment is being advocated. Thus, a nationally known psychiatrist defended lobotomy with the words, 'I just know what the brain looks like after a series of shocks — and it's not very pleasant to look at'.[81] As one neurologist has pointed out, it is ironic that while neurologists struggle to prevent any spontaneous convulsions occurring in people with epilepsy, psychiatrists are deliberately inducing multiple convulsions and claiming that it is beneficial.[82]

It is very difficult to come to an objective conclusion about the value of ECT where there are such widely differing viewpoints. Patients sometimes ask for it, and though such requests often come from 'sick role' people who want to avoid taking responsibility for themselves or from very desperate individuals (like Karen from Chapter 2) who are searching for an instant solution, there are those who say that it has helped them. A number of explanations can be put forward to account for ECT's apparently beneficial effects in some cases.

The most obvious conclusion to be drawn from Breggin's account is that ECT works quite simply by obliterating, temporarily or permanently, the memory of whatever has been causing the distress. Whether or not one can legitimately call this a cure is open to debate, and if underlying issues have not been resolved, repeated rounds may be necessary to maintain the improvement.

It has also been suggested that ECT works by relieving the guilt that is often a factor in depression: after being so thoroughly punished, a patient may be able to allow her/himself to feel better. Others have explained its effects along behavioural lines: patients who are given a treatment that they find frightening and unpleasant if they behave in certain ways (looking miserable, complaining etc.) quickly learn to behave differently in order to avoid this treatment, leading staff to believe that ECT has helped them.

There may also be a powerful placebo effect — i.e., as with

211

insulin coma therapy, the ritual, attention, and expectations surrounding the treatment may be more important than the treatment itself. Support for this theory comes from the story of the hospital whose machine, unknown to the staff, was broken and had not been delivering a current for two years; no one had noticed any difference in the results.[83]

Such useful effects as ECT does seem to achieve tend to be short-lived. One review article notes, 'it has long been accepted that its high relapse rate is one of the most serious limitations of ECT',[84] although very few studies include follow-up periods. One that did so, at Northwick Park Hospital in London, found that severely depressed patients who were given ECT did do better than a comparison group who were only given simulated ECT, but that at reassessment one month and six months later the difference between the two groups had disappeared.[86] More definite evidence of ECT's value has still to emerge, mainly because most of the hundreds of studies on it have failed to reach acceptable standards of reliability. 'ECT *may* be an effective treatment for all the conditions for which psychiatrists believe it to be useful, but even after forty years of use the gulf between the beliefs about ECT and proof of its effectiveness remains wide.'[86]

The strongest argument for its use seems to be in those rare situations where depression is so severe (involving slowed-down bodily functions, inability to eat, and so on) as to be life-threatening. ECT can, for whatever reason, jolt patients out of this dangerous state remarkably quickly, and where the stakes are so high the risks may be justified, although the authors of the Northwick Park Study concluded that 'many depressive illnesses, even if severe, may have a favourable outcome with intensive nursing and medical care even if physical treatments are not given'. However, the use of ECT is by no means confined to such cases, although exact figures on the proportion of patients who receive it are impossible to find. (None of the recent reviews have included this information among the wealth of other data.) Professor Anthony Clare has written:

It is easier to give a course of ECT than to explore a patient's social and personal circumstances. It is easier to recommend ECT than to patiently tease out complex factors such as occupational stress, marital difficulties, personal doubts, sudden bereavement, and financial anxieties. It is easier for a psychiatrist, overwhelmed by sheer number of patients, to reach for the ECT machine than to resort to more time-consuming and difficult approaches. And, because it is easier, ECT is a much abused and over-used method of treatment.[87]

Anti-depressants and lithium have not attracted the same amount of attention from non-official sources, probably because their side-effects do not seem to be so serious. It is worth noting, though, Breggin's argument that they, like the major tranquillizers, work by affecting all neuronal activity in a potentially very damaging way. He also argues strongly against the notion that there are specific remedies for specific forms of mental distress, pointing out that for depression, lithium, ECT, and anti-depressants are all recommended, plus major tranquil-lizers for agitated depression and minor tranquillizers for anxiety in depression. (Since few psychiatric patients, unless they are manic, are particularly happy, it is possible to argue a case for using any or all of these treatments on any patient — and indeed this is what tends to happen to patients who stay around long enough.) However it may be that the benefit/draw-back ratio is more favourable with anti-depressants and lithium, although an assessment of their true worth is very hard to make at the present time.

ANTI-DEPRESSANTS

Most cases of depression (which, it has been estimated, account for around 10 to 20 per cent of surgery visits)[88] are treated by GPs without being referred on to the psychiatric team. Anti-depressants are the commonest treatment offered. It is not known exactly how they work, but they are generally believed to be most effective in severer cases. Their value in milder depres-sion, where they are widely prescribed, is less certain, especially since many of these episodes lift of their own accord in about three weeks — the same length of time that it takes for the drugs to start working.

As always, the benefits of these drugs have to be weighed against the disadvantages. The MAOI group are used less often because of their potentially dangerous interaction with some foods. The more recent 'second generation' anti-depressants are very similar to the longer established tricyclic groups and the tricyclics in their turn are chemically very similar to the major tranquillizers and share some of the same side effects (sedation, concentration difficulties, confusion especially in the elderly, dry mouth, blurred vision, reduced sexual interest, and so on), although tardive dyskinesia does not seem to be a risk. The tricyclics are particularly dangerous in overdose, accounting for about 400 deaths (or about 15 per cent of all drug deaths) a year.[89]

The anti-depressants are not popular or pleasant drugs to take, and in fact an estimated 50 per cent of people fail to complete the prescribed course.[90] Some people experience withdrawal symptoms (stomach cramps, depression, restlessness, etc. from the tricyclics; headaches, shivering, and panic from the MAOIs) especially after taking the drugs for longer periods of time. The symptoms can be mistaken for a re-emergence of the original problem and lead to further prescribing.

LITHIUM

Lithium is believed to be very effective in some cases of manic-depression — a condition where a person suffers from severe mood swings, becoming either very high or very low or sometimes both in turn. It can be used to abort a manic episode, although major tranquillizers do this job more quickly. Mostly, though, it is used prophylactically, i.e. to prevent further episodes occurring, and may be taken for many years or even for life. Lithium is said to reduce the frequency and/or severity of manic episodes, although its value in preventing depression is less certain. One authority regrets 'the general hesitation about administering drugs to children and to inmates in penal or ward institutions' since proof of 'lithium effects on periodic aggressiveness is so solid'.[91]

Lithium was initially said to produce 'no unwanted effects on mood or behaviour'.[92] In fact there are a number of possible side-effects, ranging from mild sleepiness or nausea to more serious hand tremor, kidney damage, muscle weakness, and confusion. The latter may be a sign that the lithium level in the blood, which has to be monitored very carefully by regular blood tests, is too high and needs regulating to avoid the risk of intoxication. There is some evidence of a withdrawal syndrome in the form of a recurrence of the original symptoms, which could lead to patients being persuaded to re-start lithium and take it for longer than necessary.[93]

HOW DRUGS AND ECT ARE USED IN PRACTICE

Textbooks on psychiatry give very little idea of how drugs and ECT are actually used in day-to-day practice. Only about one-fifth to one-sixth of in-patients and day-patients will be on no drugs at all.[94, 95] (The commonest drugs in psychiatric hospitals are laxatives, taken by about one-quarter of patients to combat the constipating side-effects of the rest of their medication.)[96] Many will be taking several at once in potentially dangerous combinations or 'cocktails' — this is known as polypharmacy — or in very high doses. GPs have frequently been criticized for irrational prescribing of minor tranquillizers and anti-depressants, and 'evidence is growing of polypharmacy, inadequate or excessive doses, and incorrect prescribing in psychiatric hospitals'[97] as well, according to one survey. It discovered, among other things, that nearly one-half of the patients who were on medication were taking two or more drugs; that minor tranquillizers were frequently prescribed together with major tranquillizers and anti-depressants, although since the major tranquillizers and some of the anti-depressants have a sedative effect this should be unnecessary; one-third of the patients on major tranquillizers were taking two at once, by mouth and by slow-release injection, despite evidence that this increases the risk of tardive dyskinesia; one-half of the patients on major tranquillizers were also receiving anti-Parkinsonian drugs to reduce the side-effects, although this increases the severity of tardive dyskinesia, (reducing the dose of the major tranquillizers is a safer measure that should be tried first); 40 per cent of patients on major tranquillizers did not have a diagnosis of schizophrenia, while nearly one-half of the patients on anti-depressants did not have a diagnosis of clinical depression — and so on. A previous survey had found that 40 per cent of patients with problems of a known physical origin such as dementia were taking major tranquillizers,[98] which would hardly have enhanced whatever degree of mental functioning they still retained.

As these findings suggest, the decision to try someone on a particular treatment is often not based on the officially recommended indications, but is a function of the staff's desperation or the length of time the patient has been around. As one writer admitted in an unusual burst of frankness, the policy for chronic patients is that 'everybody is tried with everything worth trying as a new effective drug'.[99] Caffeine and nicotine from constant tea-drinking and cigarette-smoking, which punctuate the day in institutional life, form a background to the prescribed drugs.

The Royal College of Psychiatrists has published guidelines for the use of ECT: who should make the decision that it should be given, what staff should be present in the room, and so on. However, a recent report to the college indicates that actual practice falls far short of these recommendations:

> Twenty-seven per cent of clinics had serious deficiencies such as low standards of care, obsolete apparatus, unsuitable buildings, and could not easily be brought to a satisfactory standard; included in these were 16 per cent with very serious shortcomings: ECT was given in unsuitable conditions, with a lack of respect for the patient's feelings, by staff who were ill-trained, including some who consistently failed to induce seizures. . . . About half of the junior staff received only minimal training, i.e. someone usually not much more experienced had shown them how to press the button. . . . About 40 per cent of the clinics did not regularly maintain their apparatus. . . .[100]

Much of this use of drugs and ECT can more properly be described as treatment for the doctor, the staff, or the ward than for the individual patient. Heavier sedation when there is a shortage of staff obviously makes the ward easier to manage, but is not necessarily in the best interests of the patients. With outpatients, writing a prescription is the accepted way for a GP or psychiatrist to bring a consultation to an end and, if necessary, fend off a problem that the doctor does not know how to deal with. As one woman in a survey on minor tranquillizers said, 'I feel that, essentially, when a doctor prescribes a pill for me, it's to put *him* out of *my* misery'.[101] In the same way, the standard response to a report in the ward round that Mrs Smith or Mr Jones is no better is to suggest a change in the medication and move on to the next patient. This game can be played literally for years, so that long-standing patients may have been tried on 20 or 30 different drugs in various combinations with little or no improvement in their condition. In the short term this is far easier than trying to unravel the complex mixture of psychological and social factors that contribute to mental distress, but as MIND points out, 'no treatment programme will be successful unless it offers the patient the support he needs to come to terms with his personal crisis'.[102] MIND also says, 'For most people suffering from depression, drugs and ECT are often the only forms of help offered by the NHS'.[103] This is equally true for other forms of mental distress.

All patients, except for a very few of those who are compulsorily detained in hospital, have the right to refuse treatment, and before treatment can begin they must give legally valid consent to it. The law on this issue is complicated, but involves three main elements:

(a) patients must be given information on the nature and purpose of the treatment and any serious side effects, though this need not be an exhaustive list of every possible risk;

(b) they must be able to understand the nature and purpose of the treatment;

(c) their consent must be given without undue force, persuasion, or influence being brought to bear on them.[104]

In my experience (but confirmed by others as well) these conditions are frequently, even routinely, disregarded. Decisions about medication are made by the staff during the ward round, and patients may simply be presented with the pills at the evening drug round without being involved in any discussion about the matter. Patients who take it upon themselves to warn others about possible side-effects are not popular with the staff. ('We've just managed to get Angela to take her lithium and now John has told her that it might make her put on weight.') As we have seen, doctors are unaware of many of the more serious hazards for which evidence has been presented in this chapter, but they frequently fail to pass on even such information as is well known to them — for example, the risk of tardive dyskinesia with major tranquillizers. One survey found that half of all ECT patients felt that they had not had the treatment explained to them properly beforehand,[105] while another noted that 'discussion of risks was often only brief'.[106] There are also instances where a minority of harassed and demoralized nurses do use 'undue force, persuasion, or influence' on patients; for example, threatening them with transfer to a long-stay ward or to the local Victorian asylum if they do not take their medicine. Perhaps most influential is the combination of the whole hospital set-up where the psychiatrists and staff so clearly wield the power and make the decisions with the tendency of the average psychiatric patient to believe that doctors and other experts know what is best for him or her. This means that it is both difficult and comparatively rare for patients to question or refuse the treatment that has been prescribed. In addition, the very nature of sedative drugs can prevent patients complaining about side effects. The passive indifferences and unawareness that tardive dyskinesia sufferers display towards their bizarre movements has been noted by several researchers.

Some of these points were illustrated in the stories of the patients we met in earlier chapters. Elaine was the classic example of someone who was tried on everything (major tranquillizers, minor tranquillizers, ECT, lithium, and both types of anti-depressants) over a fifteen-year period in an attempt to solve her problems — everything, that is, except a move away from the medical approach itself. Sam's cancer phobia was actually made worse by his medication, since the side effects just gave him more physical symptoms to worry about; ECT was tried as a last resort, although he was highly anxious rather than clinically depressed. John didn't know why he had been prescribed anti-depressants as soon as he got in touch with his feelings about his father's death, nor did it occur to him to ask what they were for or decline to take them; he just went along with what the doctor ordered. The 'sick role' patients collected a whole chemist's shop of pills between them as the staff became increasingly desperate. Jenny Clark was put on a very high dose of major tranquillizers immediately upon her admission, although at that point she was bewildered and upset rather than irrational, and it could be argued that she fell into the category of patients who do best without these drugs. The powerful sedatives prevented her from working through and making sense of what had happened to her, but when she protested she was held down and injected. The resulting side-effects (blank face, shuffling walk, and stiff movements) were deeply distressing to her, her family, and the other patients on the ward. Mary, who had been sexually abused as a child, did not know she was to be put on medication until it was handed to her from the drug trolley. She was given no explanation as to what it was for or what side effects she might experience and was too unassertive to ask, besides being intimidated by the threats directed at other patients who tried to refuse their medication. Nor did she ask for or receive full information about the effects of ECT, although several years later there were still gaps in her memory. It took her three years, during which she suffered severe withdrawal symptoms, to come off her tablets and lose the weight she had gained while she was on them.

However, it is two of the less obvious side effects of physical treatments in psychiatry that are perhaps the most damaging. One has already been discussed in Chapter 2; it is the fact that unless great care is taken, these treatments convey the message that the person who is prescribed them is sick or crazy, and by implication that the relatives who are not receiving them play no part in the problem, and that socioeconomic factors are irrelevant. In this way the sick role is entered, the treatment barrier is set up, and the whole Rescue game begins. Even in more enlightened settings where counselling and psychotherapy are used, these hidden messages operate to contradict and undermine whatever other therapeutic work is undertaken.

The other serious side effect is the fact that the existence of this huge range of drugs, coupled with the power and influence of the drug industry, blocks the development and use of alternative approaches to mental distress. MIND again:

> There would be less need for drugs like major tranquillizers if there were more social work support and other vital community-based services available for patients and their families and it is a matter for concern that the development of new drugs dominates research into methods of coping with the causes and consequences of mental disorder.[107]

One psychiatrist comments that the major tranquillizers have been used 'not as an *adjunct* to psychological treatment . . . but as an *alternative* to such care'.[108] Teaching people relaxation, yoga, and stress reduction techniques would reduce the need for minor tranquillizers. Providing wards with soundproof rooms equipped with cushions and punchbags for pent-up patients (and indeed staff) to let out their frustrations would be an alternative to sedation. Perhaps the major casualty of the drug-oriented approach is psychotherapy, which requires a large investment of time and skill, and comes a very poor second to the attractions of the instant chemical solution.

Pioneers of different approaches have found that physical treatments come to assume a much less important role. A consultant in a community-based team which had moved towards a more social and psychotherapeutic model found

> a very dramatic decline in the use of ECT . . . it went down almost to vanishing point. I wasn't quite sure why. Because I don't think at the time my attitude had changed, that much, to ECT, I still saw it as something that was useful in the right circumstances. But those circumstances didn't seem to be arising so much. I guess people were being seen earlier, they were being helped in better ways at an earlier stage. Because nobody gets very seriously depressed overnight, they've been getting like that for months. The other thing we looked at that changed was the use of depot neuroleptics [i.e. major tranquillizers given by slow-release injection]. We had a group of people that we sort of inherited that had been on depot neuroleptics for quite a while, and the use of those went down by 60 per cent over a year . . . That's not to say we never used drugs, because sometimes we did, but it was a lot less than it would otherwise have been.[109]

The Transactional Analysis approach to schizophrenia, as we saw in Chapter 4, does not use drugs at all.

What would benefit Britain's psychiatric patients most is not the development of new wonder-drugs at vast cost, but the provision of jobs, decent housing, cheaper transport, child-care facilities so that mothers could take up work outside the home if they wanted, training in counselling for GPs, and many other measures which could usefully be financed out of the drug industry's massive profits. It can be shown that the dramatic improvements in physical health over the last 150 years were largely brought about not by medical intervention, although of course this does have a role to play, but by a higher standard of living, better sanitation and nutrition, and so on. The steep decline in tuberculosis-related deaths and in child mortality from scarlet fever, diphtheria, whooping cough, and measles had begun long before effective drug treatment for these ailments was available.[110] A similar revolution in the nation's mental health could be brought about by implementing the measures outlined above. In the absence of such reforms, it is not surprising to find that physical treatments in psychiatry are given more often to those members of society who are least powerful and suffer most from social and economic deprivation: women, the poor, the working-class, the mentally handicapped, and ethnic minorities. However, as long as the significance of the predictable cycles of opinion to which physical treatments in psychiatry are subject is ignored, the myth that the answer lies in medical intervention can be maintained, very much to the advantage of the medical profession and the drug industry.

Not everyone subscribes to this myth. One victim of minor tranquillizer addiction said, 'It seems that the drug companies make huge profits out of suppressing symptoms. . . . In my opinion these companies are merely legalized pushers.'[111] Indeed Braithwaite draws some interesting parallels between the legal and the illegal drug trade. Although 'people who foster dependence on illicit drugs such as heroin are regarded as among the most unscrupulous pariahs of modern civilization' while 'in contrast, pushers of licit drugs tend to be viewed as altruistically-motivated purveyors of a social good', he points out that in fact some of today's most powerful drug companies owe their existence to enormous profits built up between the wars from illegal trading in opium, morphine, and heroin.[112] He quotes a provocative paper which argues that many of the popular beliefs about the illegal drug trade — that it is a huge, elaborate organization crossing international boundaries; that power brokers who are concerned only with maximizing their enormous profits corner all supplies of the drug; that there is a distribution hierarchy with faceless men in some Eastern country at the top, importers and agents in between, and pushers, whose main job is to ensure that the greatest number of consumers use as much of the drug as they can afford, at the bottom; that there is a deliberate, profit-motivated creation of a need which is detrimental to the consumer and society as a whole; that bribery and corruption and other ruthless measures occur during distribution — that all these actually apply more accurately to the legal drug industry than to the illegal one.[113] In fact, the statistics for illegal drugs (274 deaths associated with the use of opiate-related drugs and cocaine in 1984)[114] seem relatively benign in comparison with some of the consequences of prescribed drugs. This is not to say that the use of heroin and other hard drugs is a good thing — it is dangerous and destructive. Nevertheless a cynic might say that the main disadvantage of illegal drugs from the official point of view is that they do not bring in a handsome income for the government, although they do provide a very useful focus of righteous indignation away from the far more serious consequences of the various legal drug trades (including alcohol and nicotine). Governments see no irony in decrying the former while supporting the interests of the latter. It was the Reagan administration, with its 'Say No' campaign against hard drugs, that under pressure from the pharmaceutical industry withdrew the legal requirement for information leaflets to be included with all prescriptions for minor tranquillizers.

SUMMARY

One writer quotes an East African tribesman who claimed to have special expertise with psychotic patients. 'I am able to cure mads. I order the patient tied and placed upon the ground. I then take a large rock and pound the patient on the head for a long time. This calms them and they are better.'[115] Some readers may detect parallels with the use of physical treatments in contemporary western psychiatry.

So, are these treatments a genuine advance on the emetics, rotatory chairs, and so on of the nineteenth century? My personal answer is a qualified 'yes' in theory, but a regrettable 'no' in practice.

The qualifications to the 'yes' should by now be obvious. Drugs and ECT are not the miracle cures that drug companies and doctors sometimes claim and that patients sometimes hope and ask for. 'Drugs are tamed poisons';[116] they all have potential side-effects and their usefulness depends on balancing the risks against the benefits in each individual case. In psychiatry, unlike in general medicine, there is no such thing as a physical treatment that cures a particular condition, nor is it known precisely how any of these treatments work. They were all discovered by accident, and although, in the words of one psychiatrist, 'such is the stuff of advance in many medical disciplines . . . when all advances are made in this way it is fair to doubt the scientific status of the subject'.[117] Moreover, many of them can, in certain circumstances, actually cause the problems that they are supposed to relieve. The most that they can claim to do is reduce some of the symptoms, although here again the pros and cons have to be carefully weighed against each other.

If ECT reduces the pain of events only by helping the patients to forget them, or if tranquillizers make people able to handle their emotions only by leaving them with no emotions to handle, then talk of a 'cure' becomes rather ironical. In that sense, after all, death 'cures' everything.[118]

Nevertheless they can play a useful role as part, but only part, of the help that is offered to people in mental distress. These people may wish to make an informed choice that, say, they want to use minor tranquillizers to tide them over a crisis, or that the side-effects of major tranquillizers are a lesser disruption to everyday life than hearing voices, or that anti-depressants will help to keep them going while they uncover the roots of their distress in counselling.

In practice, as we have seen, physical treatments are used in a far from ideal way. The same quality that makes them potentially more valuable than rotatory chairs and so on, i.e. their ability to affect the mind, also makes them potentially more dangerous. A genuine straitjacket is to be preferred to a chemical one in that it does at least leave your mind free, and its effects end when it is untied. The cumulative side-effects of drugs and ECT as they are used at present — the physical damage to individual patients, the 'sick role' implications that they carry, the reluctance to consider psychological and social factors and approaches — have, in my opinion, far outweighed the benefits.

Medical model psychiatry needs to use and claim success for physical treatments in order to maintain its credibility. Paradoxically, it is this same need and the resulting overuse and misuse of physical treatments that has made them into far more of a liability than an asset. Only a move away from the medical model approach will enable physical treatments to find a limited but genuinely useful role for themselves as one aspect of the help that some mentally distressed people may choose to receive.

10

Changing the system

We have discussed two partial answers to the question of why, if much of psychiatry has such a damaging effect on the people it claims to be helping, it stays the way it is. The training that the various professions receive is one factor, and this training is itself one result of a second factor, i.e. the enormously influential position that the medical model approach has carved out for itself over the last 200 years, very much in the interests of the powerful medical profession and the even more powerful drug industry. Further clues can be found by looking at what happens when people working within the system attempt to challenge it. 'If you want to know how things really are, try to change them.'[1]

Of a number of accounts of reform in psychiatric institutions, perhaps the most fascinating and readable is Jan Foudraine's *Not Made of Wood*.[2] Dr Foudraine is a Dutch psychiatrist who was trained in the traditional way.

> Of my time as a clinical medical student I can only recall that I struggled with mounting admiration through the thick tomes written by clinical psychiatrists on 'psychoses'. What the various authors had committed to paper by way of expert knowledge, observations, minute and subtle descriptive accounts, and how they larded these with a great mass of profound philosophical thinking and theorizing, often made my head reel. I nearly became convinced that . . . my intelligence was too limited to enable me to cope with such profundities. As a clinical medical student I helped to collect 'schizophrenics' from the various wards, whom we . . . then interrogated about their delusions, hallucinations, mental blocks, thought-

disturbances, and whatever else had to be investigated. In short, we would inquire how their 'craziness' was getting on; and they (who had gone through all this before) would show us how crazy they were. . . . Tranquillizers had made their appearance; I prescribed them. From time to time I pressed the button of an electroshock apparatus.[3]

Gradually he moved away from the belief that the psychotic (crazy) person was qualitatively different and suffering from some kind of disease, although 'I discovered that this latter idea was a delusion entertained by a lot of psychiatrists and very much harder to tackle than the "fantasies" of people I met in the psychiatric institutions.'[4] Appointed to a small ward for chronic schizophrenic patients in America, he began to try to understand and encounter them as 'people like you and me. . . . Just people in profound, existential need, dire need . . . and for that reason all the more human';[5] and to confront and change the ward system within which they had lived for up to twenty-five years. Although these patients had more chronic and serious problems than most, the issues that arose for the staff and the psychiatric institution itself are the same everywhere and the following extracts will focus on these aspects of the reforms.

On his arrival, Foudraine found a very traditional set-up. The staff hierarchy descended from the top ranks, who issued the general decisions and orders and were furthest away from the patients, down to those with most patient contact, the low-salary, low-status nurses, while right at the bottom of the hierarchy were the patients themselves. The chronic and apparently hopeless condition of these patients had led to profound demoralization on the part of the lower-status staff, who, perhaps as a way of coping with their despair, had lapsed into what Foudraine calls 'physical disease ideology', the belief that the patients were suffering from incurable physical illnesses and that nothing much could be done for them anyway. The staff spent as much time as possible with each other behind the closed doors of the nurses' office. The layout of the shabby and badly designed ward contributed to the generally depressing atmosphere. The whole approach encouraged passivity on the part of the patients, who had their meals served, clothes sorted, and pocket money doled out by the staff.

After some months Foudraine started to introduce reforms designed to give the patients more responsibility, and 'from that moment on the chaos was complete'. It will not be a surprise, recalling what happened when Jeanette was challenged (Chapter 3), to hear that the patients resisted extremely strongly. The following scene resulted when they were asked to help with the cooking:

> Isabel saw the grill and talked and screamed about knowing a policeman named Mr Grill. Sandy said she did not have enough strength to help and got up and took a large can of beans and threw them on the floor . . . Lesley said she would pour the tea in the salad and Cathy stopped her. Lesley then ate an onion (skin and all), etc., etc.

What is of particular interest, though, is how these changes highlighted the need of the *staff* to carry on in the traditional way. As their roles changed, they experienced extreme anxiety about what they should be doing instead. 'Again and again they would come to me and ask: "What should I do? I don't know what I should do anymore" . . . The loss of their former role was such an enervating experience that for a time they felt themselves and their function to be without meaning or purpose.' The temptation to step in as before was sometimes overwhelming. 'They simply did not believe that these activities could be taken over by patients; and it became obvious as time went on that *they themselves were unwilling to give up* a great part of them.' One of the nursing assistants, Mrs Care, who had taken over one of the most difficult patients when her daughter left home was a typical example:

> Lesley's job is to clean up the living room. She stands in the middle of the room, holding the dust mop and flapping it around childishly. Mrs Care is beside her coaxing her on without much conviction. Lesley keeps thrusting the mop into Mrs Care's hand and Mrs Care tried to give it back to her again. Mrs Care clearly feels quite miserable; and I am told she has recently become very depressed.[6]

Other staff were afraid of losing their jobs if the patients became too independent.

It was even worse when the nurses were asked to take a further step towards breaking down the staff/patient barrier and stop wearing uniforms. 'The white uniform was for me the crowning glory of my career. I had done all my training, I had got my diploma, for this.'[7] The loss of status and security that was implied was too much for many of the staff to bear. At times they hated Foudraine, and he learned later that they had held secret meetings in which they planned to resign en bloc.

When Foudraine insisted that the patients should take a share of responsibility for the cleaning, 'the result was a ward in a state of total squalor', and this plunged Foudraine into conflict with the wider institution. The attitude of the rest of the hospital had up till then been characterized by amused tolerance. 'They used to call us "that crazy bunch at Rose Cottage" . . . sometimes they would say, "He's crazy. Has he cured anybody yet?".'[8] However, a hygiene inspector who toured the ward during its worst stage of 'thoroughgoing pollution' took a more serious view, and for a while the whole hospital came under threat of closure.

In fact, this crisis seemed to serve as a turning point for the ward staff who, faced with the threat from outside, started to rally round in defence of the new regime. Further reforms were introduced, although not without difficulty. There was the breaking of the rule that patients should never carry keys, and the decision that they could take responsibility for ordering the drugs. One nurse described her initial reaction to this:

At Hillside [her previous place of work] nobody touched the medicine cabinet but me. But then the head nurse came and said, 'No, Cathy will do that'. Cathy then came and ordered the drugs. It made me feel kind of useless. I thought: Here I go through three years of nurse's training and I can't even order drugs.[9]

Then there was the decision to make the medical notes and the daily nursing reports public, so that patients could listen and, if necessary, add and correct.

An even more radical step was to banish medical words like hospital, patient, doctor, sick, illness, and so on, and hopefully eradicate with them the medical model view that seemed to Foudraine to be keeping both staff and their charges so stuck.

I forbade the 'patients' to use this language anymore and proposed calling them 'students' . . . Rose Cottage I described as a 'school for living'; and Julia was instructed to make a large board with the words THIS IS A SCHOOL FOR LIVING and to hang it on the wall of the room. The 'Nursing Office' sign we changed to 'Educational Office'. I asked the staff to go along with the experiment and named them 'assistant educators'. I told the new-born 'students' that the name 'hospital' had been an especially unhappy choice and made my apology for this. In short, I told them that we in Rose Cottage had come together in a 'school for living' where they, the students, could learn what had gone wrong with their lives and how things could be made different. . . . I told my baffled group of newly baptized 'students' and the personnel that there was no such thing as 'mental illness', that it did not exist, and that it would be better for them to regard themselves as *ignorant* about themselves and the forming of relationships with others.[10]

Although this idea was far from welcome to many of the 'students' and some of the 'educators', it gradually took hold and made a dramatic change to the atmosphere of the ward.

The whole experience took two years, and by the end the results were remarkable. All the patients, hitherto regarded as dangerous and incurable, had made dramatic improvements, and several were able to leave hospital after decades in psychiatric institutions and lead relatively independent lives outside. The changes on the ward were no less startling. Not all the staff could cope with it; Mrs Care, who had looked after Lesley, asked to be transferred, and a senior doctor commented rather sourly,

Patients started coming into the nursing office in Rose Cottage as the years progressed and it made me feel uncomfortable. During the five minutes that I'm over there I have noticed that the staff seem to be more interested in dealing with and relating to the patients than in giving me and the supervisor a report. The staff seemed to be enjoying the job too much.

But others said,

Two years ago the people here used to bawl and shout a great deal, smash things up rather a lot, and there were frequent fights, too. The 'cold wet sheet pack' was an automatic procedure. . . . We can express warmer feelings now and it seems much more genuine to me.

At one time we relied very heavily on the night supervisor, Mrs S, about what we should do, asking her for advice and that sort of thing. Now we seldom bother her with anything. . . . I think that Mrs S gets phone call after phone call from other units asking 'can we do this, can we do that?'. . . . We feel we know our patients better than anyone else and consequently we do what's beneficial.

I've noticed that I stay sitting around in Rose Cottage longer than on other wards. It has something to do, I think, with a different kind of relationship that has sprung up here between personnel and patients. . . . Patients are obviously welcome. When I go to another ward, I get involved in a pseudo-intellectual sort of conversation with the nursing personnel about problems. I notice more emotional interaction, people either like each other or hate each other's guts.

To me the patients were just vegetables. They stayed that way for about a year after our programme started. First you had to get the staff on your side: So long as we were still against you, nothing could alter. But now there's a feeling of a breakthrough. I can talk much better with everybody. How should I put it? On a different level. There's a different feeling about. In the old days we all had our jobs mapped out. It was really rather easy. Now there's something happening every minute and yet the nights are much more peaceful. . . . Now instead of patients I can see people.[11]

The barrier between staff and patient, the 'healthy' and the 'sick', had to a large extent been broken down, and the growth of the staff was parallel to, and necessary for, the growth of the patients.

It has only been possible to touch briefly on some of the main points of Foudraine's tale, which is well worth reading in full. These extracts do, however, highlight some of the universal themes of attempts to reform the psychiatric system (and systems in general). As Foudraine notes, the aims are often very similar: ' "democratizing", changing the vertical organizational structure into more horizontal forms, promoting co-responsibility and giving a bit of real encouragement to the category of people who form the lowest echelon in the institution's chain of demand.' The results are often similar too:

> More often than not the reformers are lone operators . . . and what they achieve are minimal modifications in the psychiatric institution. The reformers struggle against a mountain of opposition, and when, disillusioned or not, they eventually depart, the organization often rapidly sinks back into its bureaucratic, hierarchical, doctor-knows-best structure.[12]

The stage at which the old system is in disarray and the new one has yet to emerge seems to be the most critical. At this point, chaos and resistance is at its height and the very survival of the attempted reforms is at stake. Even winning through to the other side, as Foudraine did, is no guarantee of lasting success. It is a sad and disillusioning experience to visit a ward or hospital in the wake of a pioneer who has moved on and see how the remnants of his innovations have lingered, sanitized and absorbed into the system: the community meetings that are now largely devoted to the discussion of medication, the rule about referring to people as clients even though they are in fact treated as patients in every other respect, and so on. The system moves quickly to cover up the traces of such experiments. The consultant at one hospital where I worked had introduced a ward meeting in which all the staff and patients met together to discuss emotional and relationship issues; it was an exciting and at times moving experience. The very day after he left, a nurse who had been a key member of the group was told that he had been transferred to a different consultant's team, another nurse was moved onto night duty, while a third was forbidden to continue leading the therapy group where staff and patients shared their problems together, on the grounds that he did not have medical supervision.

Staff resistance comes from three main areas. First, and most straightforwardly, the staff need the patients quite as much as the patients need the staff, if only because their jobs depend on it. Foudraine found that by getting staff to encourage responsibility and independence in the patients, he was asking them to cut off the branch they were sitting on — a fact that was well understood by the patients. In fact he believes that in a different setting, 'a lot of the usual staff of a psychiatric institution *are indeed superfluous and so will be out of a job. . . .* if the psychiatric institution still has a future — which I doubt — there is every reason drastically to *reduce* the size of the staff, and not — as we are so often told — to increase it.'[13]

Second, the staff may need the patients to be and to continue to be patients for their own personal reasons. Foudraine's Mrs Care was apparently dealing with her women's role problems by finding a substitute daughter in one of the most helpless patients after her own daughter left home. Other factors which may make it very hard for staff to allow patients to develop into competent and confident adults include the need to maintain a sense of importance and control; to feel useful and wanted; and to avoid confronting your own fears and 'crazy' parts by locating them all in other people.

Third, there is the complicated issue of *identification with the system*. It is impossible to work within any system, the psychiatric one in this case, without to some extent becoming part of it, and thus having an investment in its continued existence. This comes about partly through the training process, and the longer and more arduous it is and the more power and status accrues to you at the end, the greater will be your investment in keeping things as they are. In psychiatry this applies most strongly to doctors, but, as Foudraine found, certainly not only to them.

At a more fundamental level individuals within the system will adopt, without always realizing it, the views of the system in which they work. Its unquestioned assumptions and values become their unquestioned assumptions and values. The medical model on which the psychiatric system is based has penetrated very deeply into the minds of psychiatric staff. Sometimes the identification is owned at a conscious level; thus, psychiatrists write books and articles in defence of a particular viewpoint (the medical model versus the psychotherapeutic model versus the social model etc.). More often, and more difficult to challenge and change, the assumptions have taken root much deeper, so that the member of staff is no longer aware that she or he is indeed making assumptions, that this view is only one of a number of possible views that she or he might hold. The assumptions have become an intrinsic part of the person's whole way of thinking — she or he '*knows*' that this is the way the world is. The phenomenon has been described by the anthropologist Evans-Pritchard: 'He cannot think that his thought is wrong.'[14] Foudraine's staff illustrated this point. For them it was — initially at any rate — *obviously* crazy to expect the patients to help with the chores. It was *obviously* ludicrous to start calling them 'students'. For many doctors it is *obvious* that patients cannot be allowed to have access to their medical files. It is *obvious* to most psychiatrists that people whom they judge to be mentally ill are in need of psychiatric treatment, and that it is a psychiatrist's duty to provide this, even if the people themselves resist it. Patients come into hospital because it is *obvious* that doctors must know what is best for them, and once in hospital it is *obvious* to most staff, patients, relatives, and members of the public that they must be mentally ill or else they wouldn't be there at all, would they?

The problem is that the more completely identification with the system occurs, the greater is the danger of losing sight of the real people within it. This is a tendency within all systems. Schools, businesses, prisons, the Church may all fall into the trap of seeing their members not primarily as human beings but as objects, whose humanity is less important than their potential as exam-passers, contract-winners, or candidates for punishment or conversion. In the psychiatric system, the danger is of seeing those who use the service as patients first and people second. Scott has described the situation thus:

> All people who work in a public service work in a psycho-political field which I term the 'System'. . . . To a greater or lesser extent staff internalize the System into their thinking and seeing and in doing so they lose their own shape as persons. To the extent that this happens we will find that they see illness and chronicity rather than the healthy parts of the patient's personality, and that they are then liable to feelings of hopelessness. They become trapped in the System.[15]

The extent to which identification has occurred is not usually apparent until (as with 'sick role' patients) there is an attempt to challenge the underlying assumptions, and then the strength of the resistance and anxiety that is stirred up, even in apparently more enlightened members of staff, gives a clue to the power of the forces one is dealing with. The danger is that if the assumptions go unchallenged, staff will inevitably act out and pass on, largely at an unconscious level, those aspects of the system which they have incorporated into their own way of thinking. Thus Foudraine's staff, with their unquestioned belief that the patients were suffering from incurable physical illnesses, behaved and treated the patients as if this was so, and the patients absorbed this belief as well and behaved accordingly. Another of the staff's unquestioned assumptions was that the patients were incapable of taking responsibility for themselves, and this contributed to a style of working that actually made the patients less responsible and more helpless. Thus, the assumptions become self-fulfilling prophecies; people who are treated primarily as patients, with all that the term implies, will come to live up to this image and the staff's beliefs will be further reinforced. The final irony is that the staff themselves fall into their own trap. As Foudraine notes, psychiatric nurses and aides *'begin gradually to react with just as much chronic schizophrenic behaviour as the patients with whom they have to deal'*.[16] In dehumanizing others, they become dehumanized themselves.

There have been a number of examples of the consequences of identification with the system in earlier chapters. For instance, we saw how staff who have never questioned their assumptions about men's and women's roles but have instead accepted them as self-evident facts about the way the world is, will draw up treatment plans that reflect and pass on these assumptions. The fact that the internalized values of the system are passed on unconsciously makes them, from the patient's point of view, particularly hard to recognize and challenge, and for that reason all the more powerful. If the messages were made explicit ('We at St John's Hospital believe that a woman's place is in the home'; 'Your treatment will be based on the assumption that your job is more important than your emotional life') then at least the patient would have a chance to evaluate them and decide whether or not she or he was in agreement. As it is disagreement has to appear in the form of unresolved symptoms — continued inability to cope with the chores, persistent panic attacks on the way to the office — which are labelled by both staff and patient as illness. The patient has been mystified — confused about the origins of her/his distress by a powerful message that has not been made explicit. Mystification on the part of the patient is the logical result of identification with the system on the part of the staff. The final result is to reinforce the tendency of patients to internalize their oppression, as the phrase goes. Instead of being enabled to locate a significant portion of their problems where they belong, in externally imposed conditions and expectations, they adopt and impose those same conditions on themselves, and the messages that they receive about being unworthy or inferior are translated into actually experiencing themselves as unworthy and inferior. Depressed housewives, for example, do not need anyone else to tell them to rush home from hospital and do the chores; they are by far their own worst enemies in this respect, often to the exasperation of their families, and yet no amount of work adds up to a feeling of self-worth and self-esteem. Similarly, men who have broken down either physically or psychologically through driving themselves too hard at work find it enormously hard to alter their lifestyle, rather than taking up the harness again far too soon in an effort to prove themselves.

The tremendous obstacles in the way of successful reform are apparent. Indeed, given the unusual combination of abilities that a potential innovator needs to possess, it is surprising that the more radical reforms ever get under way at all. In the present psychiatric set-up he (and so far they all seem to be male) will need to be a doctor, since otherwise he will not have the necessary power and status to introduce changes. His training will have steeped him in the traditional views and he will need to adhere to some form of them in order to rise up the medical hierarchy at all — more unorthodox candidates will probably not enter the profession in the first place. Having questioned and abandoned many of his basic assumptions, he must use his medical status in order to de-medicalize the system, be autocratic about imposing democracy, highly sensitive and yet able to bear the anger that will be directed towards him, and willing to risk confronting and hurting people in order to introduce a more caring and humane approach.

All this raises the important and difficult question of whether real change is in fact possible. There are two main schools of thought here, one of which advocates reform, while the other insists that nothing short of revolution will do.

Not surprisingly, the 'revolution' position is one that tends to be held by those who have experienced the psychiatric system as patients rather than as staff. Thus, the manifesto for the Psychiatric Inmates' Liberation Movement states, among other things:

We believe that psychiatry cannot be reformed, but must be abolished. . . . *We demand* the dismantling of the entire 'mental health' system by ending forced psychiatric practices, closing all psychiatric institutions, terminating all 'mental health' training programmes, dissolution of all lobby groups such as the World Psychiatric Association and national affiliations, and removing all legal, medical, and professional sanctions.[18]

This tends to be accompanied by the view that all mental health professionals are untrustworthy and damaging, however benevolent their motives are. The danger is that unless people can find a way of relating to and coming to terms with the old system and acknowledging its good aspects, the 'new' system will turn out to be very much the same as the old one but in a different guise. An example is found in extreme versions of feminism which have turned the tables by discriminating against and denigrating men.

Sympathetic as one may be to the anger and suffering that has led to such sweeping condemnations and demands, one has to remember that violent revolution tends to lead to the emergence of exactly the same situation in reverse, as the pendulum swings from one extreme to the other. Categorizing all psychiatric staff as enemies in the pay of an oppressive system is only the other side of the coin from Persecuting patients for not getting better. Insisting that mental health professionals have nothing at all to offer is the counterpart of seeing patients as the helpless Victims of disease processes.

On the other hand, as we have seen, attempts to reform the system often seem to be doomed before they even start. The point is made in a paper which discusses

> the myth of the hero-innovator: the idea that you can produce, by training, a knight in shining armour who, loins girded with new technology and beliefs, will assault his organisational fortress and institute changes both in himself and others at a stroke. Such a view is ingenuous. . . . The fact of the matter is that organizations such as schools and hospitals will, like dragons, eat hero-innovators for breakfast.[19]

And Foudraine believes that

> attempts to reform the mental hospital fundamentally have generally failed. . . . My experience has convinced me that our present psychiatric institutions are extremely difficult to reform and that we shall have to look for alternatives to them,

235

and that the training of psychiatrists and everything else that is involved in psychiatry needs a complete overhaul because they are riddled with faulty, not to say logically untenable, traditional basic assumptions.[17]

The third option, setting up private facilities outside the NHS, has been chosen by many psychotherapists and by others such as those who use the Transactional Analysis approach to schizophrenia. This has the obvious disadvantage of leaving the main system to carry on exactly the same as before, while only those with the necessary money and awareness are able to take advantage of the alternatives.

So what is the answer to this difficult problem?

I believe that to a large extent, individuals have to work out their own personal compromises according to their different temperaments, situations, and experiences. Former users of the psychiatric services are obviously in the best position to publicize the patient's point of view and to organize consumer pressure groups; relatives and organizations such as MIND can campaign for better services; many members of staff will choose to remain within the system and introduce their own ideas as far as possible, while others will decide that for them the compromises are too great and that their energies are best directed towards setting up their own private services where there are not such rigid limitations to their effectiveness. Perhaps most crucially of all, the general public, which on the whole knows extraordinarily little about psychiatry, needs to be better informed about the issues that are involved. This is partly so that they can avoid becoming victims of the psychiatric system themselves, but more importantly because for any genuine change to occur, pressure will have to come from outside the psychiatric system as well as from within it. One of the main aims of this book is to promote a greater awareness of the important issues in psychiatry among interested laypeople, and this is particularly relevant at a time of increasing public concern about the shortcomings of the community care programme.

In general terms, I believe that there is no real alternative to the slow, painful, unglamorous, and often unsuccessful process of trying to create awareness of identification with the system, or 'consciousness-raising', to use the jargon term. Frustrating and difficult as these efforts can undoubtedly be, I believe that they are the only way to achieve genuine and lasting change, because without them we will not even be aware that change is necessary and the old system will simply be carried forward into new settings, as has happened numerous times in the history of psychiatry. This is the dilemma for the community care movement at the moment. Organizational change is being imposed on the psychiatric system from above, but unless this is paralleled by a fundamental revision of attitudes in the hearts and minds of those who work in the system, real change will have eluded us once again. In other words, I am advocating reform rather than revolution, and change that starts from the revision of internal attitudes rather than from the overthrow of external conditions, while admitting that this is a slow and difficult process and perhaps even an impossible one without the added ingredient of public awareness and pressure from users of the service as well.

These themes are present in Scott's work (Chapter 4). Scott started off as a fairly traditional psychiatrist:

I myself have been through various stages in my relation with the System. First I was very much unaware of how I was contained in the System. Then largely through research I became more aware. The research concerned the relation between schizophrenic patients and their families and how the Hospital System figured in this relation. . . . In view of these findings I and my team opened up our section of the hospital to the outside world. Before any possible admission came near the hospital we saw the identified patient in the natural setting of his life and in the presence of his relatives or involved others. We created a family therapy framework in which we would usually start by demystifying our medical role in the course of making clear what we could offer and then try to get clear from the patient and his involved others what would be their commitment in this situation. Thus I actively fought the System. But at the same time I noticed that my dreams were often saying that I was in the power of the System. It was much later that I seriously took account of the fact that one was as much identified with the System if one fought it as one was by going along with its way. . . . For instance when seeing a family in crisis the family might want admission of a member whilst we, in fighting the System, saw admission as bad. In this situation the patient would be a pawn who was not treated by us, by his family, and probably not by himself either, as a human being. If we unwisely entered into this fight then the dragon of the System might appear when the family would threaten to go to a higher authority to secure what they wanted. . . . Thus we reach the problem of trying to find the *middle way.* . . . The middle way is always between polar opposites and it is always the human way.[20]

Individual systems are only cogwheels within larger ones and it is impossible to introduce real changes in the former without affecting the latter. This is as true at an individual level (thus, Elaine Jones's own psychological changes affected the whole family set-up), as at an organizational level (Foudraine's innovations brought him into conflict with the rest of the hospital). Ultimately, the system that truly radical reforms come up against is the society in which we all live, and this is what happened to Scott and his team. Taking a closer look at what happened will illustrate this point and will also demonstrate the most important and fundamental reason why the psychiatric system resists reform and remains the way it is.

In Chapter 4 we saw how Scott's reforms caused what he described as a 'bloody revolution' within the hospital, which found its very existence threatened by the fall in admission rates. Clashes with senior staff prevented nurses from being fully integrated into the crisis intervention team. Like Foudraine's staff, many of them found it very hard to cope with the de-medicalizing of their role and the handing over of more responsibility to the patients. ('Nurses who were trained to regard mental patients as sick people, and who were accustomed to helping, caring for, and comforting them in rather the same way as the physically ill, found it hard to adjust to a system whereby the patients were treated as responsible for their actions and capable of looking after their own physical needs',[21] as an investigation into the services put it.) As on Foudraine's ward, there were threats to the very existence of the team during the predictable intermediate stage of anxiety, chaos, and squalor. But because the reforms challenged not only the way the psychiatric service was run but also the whole way in which GPs, the police, relatives, and ordinary members of the public view mental illness, they came up against powerful resistance from outside the hospital as well. Lurid headlines appeared in the local and national press: 'Filth and brutality — treatment prescribed for mental patients',[22] 'Why we are brutal',[23] alongside shock-horror stories such as 'Patients had to make their beds. The patients were expected to: MAKE their own beds; WASH their own crockery; SERVE their own meals; KEEP their ward clean. If they did not serve their own meals they did not eat, and if the ward became dirty the nurses were not allowed to clean it.'[24] The *Daily Mail* carried a report on 'The doctor who was too tough. He made patients face reality',[25] and even ran a leader entitled 'The arrogance of the psychiatrists'.[26] ('Patients living rough in the hospital grounds . . . a middle-aged schizophrenic who died of physical injuries which were never fully diagnosed . . . patients and their relatives living in terror of the doctors and nurses . . . filth and chaos in the wards — it all sounds like the worst Victorian snakepit. Yet the conditions . . . were not the result of poverty or neglect within the National Health Service. They were, it seems, directly and indirectly the results of treatment methods deliberately and passionately pursued by Dr Scott and his staff', etc., etc.)

Finally the pressure of complaints led to intervention from the very highest level of the system when Sir Keith Joseph, the then Secretary of State for Health and Social Services, ordered a government inquiry into conditions at the hospital. The resulting document cleared the team of any professional negligence in the case of the patient whose death had triggered the investigation and found nothing to suggest deliberate ill-treatment or cruelty to any patient; in fact they paid tribute to Dr Scott's work and believed that the crisis intervention team should be given a fair trial. 'Napsbury Hospital owes much to Dr Scott. . . . He has functioned both as an innovator and an enabler.'[27] They did, however, criticize the conditions on some of the wards and felt that the new methods

> were pursued in an insistent and inflexible manner. The result was at times a seeming lack of compassion and of respect for the rights of patients, particularly from some of the more junior members of the team. . . . It was not so much what was done, but the way in which it was done, that in our view left Dr Scott open to legitimate criticism.

They believed that a better programme of preparation and public relations would have reduced these difficulties. The verdict was summarized with something less than total impartiality in the *Daily Express* as 'Probe calls halt to "bizarre" doctor's tough-line cure for patients',[28] while the local evening paper announced

'The harsh facts of life at Napsbury Hospital — now it's official. How doctors doled out heartbreak and misery. "This method of treatment must not be allowed to spread".'[29]

Once again, the experiences of a reformer show how important it is for staff to be able to recognize their involvement with the system in which they work. For Scott and Foudraine, losing their own battles with the hospital and wider systems would have imposed crucial limitations on their ability to help their patients in their corresponding struggles towards autonomy in their own smaller marital and family systems.

The second and even more important point highlighted by the passionate resistance of some sections of the press and the general public is the extent to which traditional medical model psychiatry is identified with society as a whole. The values of the two systems are the same; and if the assumptions of psychiatry are challenged, then the substantial proportion of society which shares these assumptions can be expected to protest very strongly. We saw in Chapter 4 how the ritual of diagnosis, officially a function performed by the psychiatrist, is in fact very often only a rubber-stamping of a decision already made by lay-people who have used their own criteria to select one person as the 'sick one' and who may become angry and abusive if the psychiatrist refuses to go along with this. One critic illustrates the point that we all demand that psychiatrists share and enforce our values with the story of an eccentric acquaintance who ended up being committed to hospital after breaching a number of social norms on an aeroplane: wearing strange clothes, raising his voice to a fellow-passenger, and so on.

> It was not some *law* that Noah broke but a social rule, something not written down in any code of justice anywhere in the United States. Thou shalt not raise thy voice in a Boeing 707. That is all Noah really did. . . . No question about it — he'd flipped his lid. . . . Yet who are these people who are making this judgement? There were no psychiatrists on the airplane. . . . Not professionals, in other words, but everyday 'normal' people, police and passengers, decided he was crazy. Which is a way of saying that we — you and I, the public — made that diagnosis. . . . Let the psychiatrist decide whether it's schizophrenia or involutional melancholia or some other arcana they suffer from. *That's* the psychiatrist's job. He confirms and refines what is fundamentally our diagnosis. He works for *us*.

. . . The mental hospital is essentially what we want it to be, and we want an institution which will take disturbing people off our hands. . . . only a change in attitude on *our* part will eliminate the need for such custodial institutions.

But the anger and abuse that a psychiatrist may meet if he refuses to go along with this role in an individual case, is even more apparent at a more general level when a whole psychiatric service refuses to go along with what the public is demanding, consciously or unconsciously, that it should supply, i.e. the unquestioning removal of certain members of society who are thereafter to be labelled as not responsible.

This gives us additional insight into the dilemma that psychiatrists face (usually unconsciously). Working with the mentally distressed can be extremely fulfilling if you feel that you are able to offer real help to those in need. However, being caught both ways — required by society to uphold its values and sweep up its debris while being faced with an enormous amount of individual suffering — is highly uncomfortable and unsatisfying. By covertly demanding that psychiatrists act as police for our problems, we mystify them and make them, in some ways, as much victims of the psychiatric system as their patients. Perhaps it is not surprising if they turn to medical jargon, physical treatments, and fifteen-minute appointments as a way of distancing themselves from this distasteful task. But more importantly, it gives a vital clue to the origin of the fundamental contradictions in medical model psychiatry: the fact that it operates on the assumption that there is a physical basis for mental illness although none has ever been found, that its treatments lack a rationale for their effects and probably cause as much disability as they cure, that while calling for increased research and resources it resolutely turns its back on cheaper and more effective methods such as crisis intervention, and so on. In the case of an individual whose symptoms are handicapping and hard to understand and yet will not go away (a woman with agoraphobia for example), one has to look deeper to discover the underlying purpose that the symptoms may be serving — (perhaps this enforced dependency is preserving the marriage). At the level of a whole system the same principle applies. Psychiatry suffers from numerous distressing symptoms: high readmission rates, low staff morale, public suspicion, inability to define basic terms like schizophrenia, low status among other doctors, and so on. The only way to make sense of the rigidity with which it resists reform despite all these problems is to expose its underlying purpose and the central paradox that leads to all the surface contradictions. In brief, *psychiatry is required to be the agent of society while purporting to be the agent of the individual; and its main function is not treatment but social control.* This theme will be explored in more detail in the next chapter.

11

Psychiatry and wider society

In the last chapter, a discussion of resistance to reform in the psychiatric system led to the conclusion that this phenomenon could only be fully understood by seeing psychiatry as serving an important underlying purpose, and to the contention that *psychiatry is required to be the agent of society while purporting to be the agent of the individual; and its main function is not treatment but social control.*

This is not a new theory. As many readers will know, a number of arguments have been put forward in support of it. One is that to give someone a psychiatric diagnosis is in fact to make a social judgement rather than the objective scientific assessment that the medical model likes to pretend. Unlike in general medicine, there are no physical tests of temperature, blood pressure, X-rays, and so on to help make the diagnosis (except for the minority of cases where, for example, a brain tumour or advanced senile dementia is involved). Despite the reams that have been written on the essential psychiatric skill of diagnosis, in the end decisions have to be made on descriptions (withdrawn manner, impulsive actions, aggressive outbursts, inappropriate affect, delusional remarks, pressure of speech, etc.) that rely heavily on the psychiatrist's own assumptions about what is normal and acceptable. How quiet do you have to be before you can be called withdrawn? How angry is aggressive? How sudden is impulsive? How unusual is delusional? How excited is manic? How miserable is depressed? The answers to all these questions are to be found not in some special measuring skill imparted during psychiatric training, but in the psychiatrist's and relatives' shared beliefs about how 'normal' people should behave (and, as we saw in Chapter 7, the selection and training of doctors means that these beliefs are likely to be pretty conservative). Additional support for the social judgement theory comes from the writings of Emil Kraepelin, the founding father of medical model psychiatry, who around the turn of the century was the first person to attempt a definition of a new illness: dementia praecox, later renamed schizophrenia. In the absence of physical causes he had to rely for his definition on descriptions of problematic behaviour, much of which consisted merely of breaking social rules and sex-role expectations:

> They do not suit their behaviour to the situation in which they are, they conduct themselves in a free and easy way, laugh on serious occasions, are rude and impertinent towards their superiors, challenge them to duels, lose their deportment and personal dignity; they go about in untidy and dirty clothes, unwashed, unkempt, go with a lighted cigar into church, speak familiarly to strangers, decorate themselves with gay ribbons. . . . In their handiwork the loss of taste often makes itself felt in their choice of extraordinary combinations of color and peculiar forms. . . . It was mentioned with very special frequency, particularly in the male sex, that children were mostly concerned who always exhibited a quiet, shy, retiring disposition, made no friendships, lived only for themselves. Of secondary importance, and more in girls, there is reported irritability, sensitiveness, excitability, nervousness, and along with these self-will and a tendency to bigotry.[1]

One famous experiment casts doubt on psychiatrists' ability to distinguish mad from sane at all, and also illustrates how powerfully a diagnostic label affects how a person and his/her behaviour is perceived. A researcher, Rosenhan, and seven other perfectly sane individuals presented themselves to twelve different American hospitals complaining of voices saying 'empty', 'hollow', and 'thud', but otherwise describing their lives exactly as they were.[2] All were admitted to hospital, where they immediately stopped complaining of the voices and behaved perfectly normally. In no case was their sanity detected by staff (although a number of patients expressed strong suspicions) and all were discharged, after varying lengths of time, with a diagnosis of schizophrenia in remission. During their time in hospital their behaviour (for example, openly taking notes on what they observed) was consistently interpreted as part of their pathology ('Patient engages in writing behaviour'). Following these results Rosenhan neatly reversed the situation by informing one hospital that a number of other false patients would be asking to be admitted during the next three months. In fact none were sent, but this did not stop the staff from wrongly identifying 41 out of 193 referrals as the false patients they had been told to expect.

There is sometimes implicit recognition of the essentially unscientific nature of diagnosis when, for example, a doctor says, 'She still seems a bit high but I wonder if that's just her personality — could someone ask her daughter what she's usually like?'. And a classic illustration is provided by perhaps the most spectacular instant cure achieved by modern psychiatry, when homosexuality was dropped as a category of mental illness from the *Diagnostic and Statistical Manual III* in 1973 and millions of people thus 'recovered' overnight. Here was a particularly clear example of a social judgement dressed up as a medical one.

In fact, psychiatric diagnosis is notoriously unreliable, as one would expect if a large element of social judgement is involved. Studies show that even experienced psychiatrists agree on a label only about 50 per cent of the time and that different hospitals tend to develop their own particular norms and usages.[3] There are international variations too; the USSR and the USA have been criticized for over-readiness to apply the diagnosis of schizophrenia, while in some pre-industrial countries even fairly extreme behaviour is tolerated without attracting a label of craziness. In any case, such diagnoses are, at the level of day-to-day patient care, of very little real use. At the culmination of most case conferences, when much learned debate has led to the conclusion that the patient is suffering from a schizo-affective something-or-other rather than a hypomanic whatever and the patient is escorted back to the ward again, no one is any the wiser as to what they should actually *do* with him or her. In contrast, a diagnostic system that included the human element might be able to come up with a formulation — that the person was suffering from, say, unresolved mourning or difficulty in separating from parents or marital problems — that would actually have practical implications for a treatment programme.

It can be argued, then, that for a psychiatrist to give someone a diagnostic label is not only not useful, it is also more a matter of passing a concealed social judgement on their behaviour than of making an objective medical assessment. However, most of the people whose stories have been recounted in this book were clearly suffering from something more than having been given a damaging and possibly inaccurate label, although this had contributed substantially to their problems and is one of the things that patients feel most harmed by. (See, for example, Mary's account in Chapter 5 of having to change jobs and avoid friends in order to shake off the stigma of having been in a psychiatric hospital.) Correspondingly, their problems stemmed from something more complex than merely having breached some social norm. In fact, it is a common failing of many writers who have been very critical of medical model psychiatry to sabotage themselves by drawing a picture that is too black-and-white, thus enabling the defenders of traditional psychiatry to point to obvious flaws in their arguments and dismiss them altogether. The argument of this book is *not* that there is no such thing as severe mental distress, nor that psychiatrists and other staff are wicked people who deliberately set out to confuse and harm their patients, nor that psychiatric treatments are universally unhelpful, nor that patients are suffering simply and solely from labelling, scapegoating, political oppression, or whatever else. My argument is, however, *that social and political factors are a crucial component of mental distress; that through being identified with the wider system of society, psychiatry shares its values and assumptions; that the psychiatric system in its turn passes on these values and assumptions by a process of identification on the part of its staff and mystification on the part of its patients; that as a result the overall effect of psychiatry, if not the conscious intent of its practitioners, is to reinforce social norms and political interests; and that since none of this is made explicit, dissent can only emerge in the form of continued symptoms on the part of the patients.* My further contention is that *social control, the maintaining of society's status quo by labelling dissent as illness, is actually the major function that wider society, consciously or unconsciously, expects and demands that psychiatry should fulfil; that while it is certainly not possible to explain all of an individual's distress in these terms, psychiatry as a whole will be able to offer genuine help to its patients struggling in their systems only to the extent that it is aware of and successful in challenging its own role in the wider system of society; and that where it fails most spectacularly (women's problems in general, schizophrenia, mental distress in ethnic minorities) is also where such factors play the most important and ignored role in the problem. My final point is that the principal mechanism by which psychiatry performs its function of social control is the use of the medical model, i.e. by propagating the myth that psychiatry is engaged in an objective, scientific enterprise to which medical science will one day produce the solutions, which gives psychiatry powerful weapons for suppressing dissent (drugs, ECT) while enabling its true purpose to be concealed.*

Much of this has been implicit in this book so far. While we have not seen examples of card-carrying communists or declared anarchists drugged into submission, what we have found is a number of people who are in conflict with the small systems (marriages, families, workplaces, sex roles) within which they live — systems which are cogwheels within the larger system of society and are microcosms of its values. In the words of Mary (Chapter 5), 'The whole system is that you've got to conform, but when you think about it, the ones in here are non-conformists.' There were, of course, other layers to their problems too, and the full personal meaning of each individual's dilemma could only be clarified by an understanding of the particular circumstances in which they found themselves and the lessons that they, as unique individuals, had drawn from them. But at another level, we saw in Chapter 5, for example, how in accepting unquestioningly society's assumptions about the role of women, psychiatry passes on these messages to its female patients, thus mystifying them about the origins of their distress ('I know I *shouldn't* be feeling like this'). One way of interpreting the depressed housewife's continued inability to cope with the chores is that she has, at an unconscious level, decided to go on strike in protest at the conditions under which she is expected to live. Her symptoms are the only way she can say 'No' to the role assigned to her by her family, at one level, and by society in general at another level (and also to that part of herself that identifies with these standards). It became apparent that in such cases the family's request to the hospital is not just 'Make her happy again' but, covertly, 'Make her happy to fit in with the role that we think women ought to have', and the covert response of the hospital is 'We'll try to do that; and if we can't, we'll at least make sure that she doesn't question it'. This is followed up with powerful sedative drugs which further reduce her ability to think and function autonomously while purporting to be the medical cure for the problem that has been diagnosed as an illness called depression. Once again, I emphasize that this is not the conscious intent of either party; the family are genuinely concerned and the hospital staff sincerely believe they are doing their best to help. However, it is by this kind of process of labelling dissent as an illness suffered by the individual that psychiatry can be said to be acting as an agent of social control.

We can see the same process at work in the stories of women whose problems take a different form. One way of understanding the dilemma that Angela, the young anorectic woman in Chapter 5, faced, is to say that she had at some level decided to go on hunger strike in protest at the conflicting demands placed on her as a young woman. The 'hunger strike' analogy has been expanded by Susie Orbach in her book of the same name.[4]

> Like the hunger striker, she has taken as her weapon a refusal to eat. Like the suffragettes at the turn of the century in the United Kingdom or the political prisoners of the contemporary world, she is giving urgent voice to her protest. . . . Her self denial is in effect a protest against the rules that circumscribe a woman's life.

Orbach also indicates the wider political processes that form the background to a culture where eating disorders are epidemic. She points out that with the growth of the consumer society over the last twenty-five years, where objects are valued not so much for their usefulness but as symbols of status, power, wealth, or sexuality, women's bodies have increasingly been used to sell everything from cars to soft drinks.

> The sexuality of women's bodies becomes split off and reattached to a host of commodities reflective of a consumer culture. . . . For women themselves, the body has become a commodity within the marketplace or, as I have suggested elsewhere, their own commodity, the object with which they negotiate the world. . . . Women are encouraged to see their bodies from the outside, as if they were commodities.

She suggests that it is no coincidence that the obsession with slimness began

248

just at that moment in history when women were demanding to be taken more seriously in the workplace and, in the language of the 1970s, 'demanding more space'. Body maintenance, body beautiful, exercise and the pursuit of thinness are offered as valued arenas for concern precisely at the moment when women are trying to break free of such imperatives.

Again we can see how psychiatric treatment which focuses solely on weight gain and imposes a strict feeding programme is, in effect, mystifying the young woman by conveying the message that the whole problem lies in her 'illness'. It is she who has the difficulty, and she who must adjust. Denied the right to negotiate about conditions, continuing symptoms become her only means of protest.

Similar themes were traced in the stories of the men in Chapter 6, most of whose problems consisted of an inability to deal with their feelings in the accepted masculine way, something that starts to be seen as a serious problem when it begins to interfere with the central male function of holding down a job. This was true of Edward, the bank manager who had a breakdown, David, the business executive with ulcers, and Jim, whose anxiety symptoms interfered with his work both for the gas board and on his market stall. Although there was an individual flavour to all of their problems, at a more general level their dilemmas centred round an inability to subordinate their personal lives, feelings, and standards to the demands of their jobs. We also saw in Chapter 6 how the identification with the belief that a man's most important role is to have a job and be a provider leads to such devastating psychological consequences for unemployed men, who find themselves in a particularly vicious trap. Deprived of the means from which they have been taught to derive their identity and self-esteem, they are at the same time blamed for being out of work by those sections of society who find it more comfortable to believe that unemployment is a personal failing rather than a political policy. Yet if they dare to stop banging their heads against the brick wall of rejected job applications and find alternative ways of making life enjoyable and meaningful, they invite accusations of living a life of leisure and luxury at the taxpayer's expense — as though there is some rule that unemployment has to be experienced as punitive, depressing, and shameful. And indeed, from a wider point of view, this is exactly how it does need to be experienced if the many people on whose utterly monotonous and uncreative work the economy depends are to be prevented from rebelling. In the words of one worker, 'There's a lot of variety in the paint shop. You clip on the colorhose, bleed out the old color, and squirt. Clip, bleed, squirt, think; clip, bleed, squirt, yawn; clip, bleed, squirt, scratch your nose'.[5] But as long as there are economic reasons for reinforcing the traditional male attitude towards work, the exciting and creative possibilities of unemployment (distributing work fairly by means of shorter working weeks, longer holidays, part-time work, and jobsharing schemes, so that men would at last have the opportunity to become more involved in family life and child-rearing while women could correspondingly be freed to follow up jobs and interests outside the home) remain unexplored. Psychiatry contributes to maintaining the status quo, first, by reinforcing the whole traditionally masculine tendency to suppress feelings, thus helping to ensure that men do not question their roles; second, by tending to measure cure in terms of being able to get back to work; and third, by labelling those who cannot fit in with this system as 'ill'. In effect, men are punished for protesting about the conditions of their lives in the same way as women are. Unemployed men, who, as we saw in Chapter 6 have a higher rate of psychiatric breakdown, will receive the stigma of a psychiatric label in addition to the shame that they may already feel about being out of work. Again, by dispensing a form of treatment that sees the problem only in individual terms, psychiatry can be said to serve the function of disguising the results of political policy as illness and allowing it to be swept under the carpet, so that protest both on an individual and a wider level is neutralized, appearing only in the indirect form of psychological symptoms.

The group of people who use the hospital mainly to meet social or economic needs and often the 'sick role' patients too (Chapter 3) are casualties of society who find a place for themselves in the mental patient status offered by the psychiatric system. From an individual point of view this may be the best option available, but from a wider perspective it can be argued that this is one of the ways in which

the sick role becomes a convenient tool to maintain the status quo. . . . (It) permits temporary deviance from the usual role expectations. It also isolates the deviant and prevents the group formations which would be needed for fundamental social change. In this sense, the sick role cools out the opposition.[6]

Once again, I am not suggesting that social and political issues are the most important strand in every individual case, nor that it is always useful or possible to address them in treatment. Nevertheless, the argument of this book is that if you go far back enough, a clash between the needs of the individual and the values of society can always be found. The behavioural treatment of agoraphobia, for example, always involves at some point a two-hour trip to the most feared situation of all, the local Arndale Centre or shopping mall, where the unfortunate sufferer learns the hard way that even the most extreme anxiety does eventually subside. But after the fiftieth woman has described how she cannot face these places without panicking, one starts to wonder who has the problem — the patient or the planners who design these huge impersonal mausoleums.

The social control hypothesis helps to explain some of the more flagrant cases of psychiatric abuse. An example is given in a recent newspaper report[7] describing how a 22-year-old man was woken up one morning, handcuffed and compulsorily detained in psychiatric hospital for eighteen days, fourteen of them sedated, although it was later ruled that he was not suffering from a mental illness. The young man, a Mr Routley, and his father

> were at loggerheads after he failed his first-year examinations at Kent University. . . . A month earlier his mother, to whom he was very attached, had died from cancer. His father complained to the GP that Mr Routley 'loafed around the house', made no financial contribution to his keep, and would not look for a job. He also alleged that his son was violent to him and to a younger brother.

The psychiatrist who was called in had based his diagnosis on the father's report plus a brief glimpse of Mr Routley as he ran upstairs, and had then

> made arrangements for a place in a ward, for an ambulance and for police attendance, because he anticipated that Mr

Routley would resist. 'He was forcibly taken away in hand-cuffs on a stretcher, he was sat on in the ambulance and restrained. He struggled on arrival at the hospital and he was given a heavy dose of a drug to prevent further resistance. That procedure was wholly unlawful because he was not mentally ill, certainly not to justify a warrant for his detention, and certainly not a danger to himself or to others.'

Horrifying incidents like this, which certainly do occur, can only be fully understood by seeing psychiatrists as working in unconscious collusion with the values of society as exemplified by the parents. This psychiatrist presumably shared the parental view that the behaviour of a young man who loafs around the house and refuses to get a job is sufficiently incomprehensible to be labelled mad. On this model it is obvious that it is the child, the dissident in this mini-system, whose behaviour has to be suppressed by an approach that locates the whole problem in him or her in the form of an 'illness'.

There are parallels in the way that people who are diagnosed as schizophrenic enter the psychiatric system. Jenny Clark (Chapter 4) was more distressed and genuinely in need of help than the young man in the newspaper report. Yet the quite astonishing degree of blindness that most psychiatrists display in their automatic alignment with the parental/family point of view cannot be entirely explained by their need to view schizo-phrenia as a physical illness. It is possible for us perhaps to make a guess at what it is about this particular form of breakdown that constitutes such a threat and generates such an extreme response from psychiatry. A striking feature of such cases is the 'happy families' myth that is commonly presented by all parties — the child included. In the same way as depressed housewives will describe their marriages as wonderful (apart from their own selfish and irrational symptoms which spoil things) and their husbands as paragons of patience and virtue, the whole family tends to put forward an idealized picture of unfailingly close relationships, where the child grew up happy and loving although possibly just a little anxious. Such accounts are readily accepted at face value by medically-minded psychiatrists, although a very different picture emerges if psychotherapy is undertaken. The child's breakdown threatens to blow apart the myth as it applies to a particular family, but perhaps at a more general level it also threatens wider society's myth of the happy nuclear family that, like the idyllic romantic marriage, is sold to us in idealized form by everyone from politicians to washing-powder manufacturers. There is a strong political interest in promoting the nuclear family as a natural and desirable way to live, but it may well be that this way of organizing society is an intrinsically unsatisfactory way of meeting the emotional needs of the individual. It has been pointed out that with the growing impersonality of the work sphere, the family has been faced with the intolerable burden of meeting nearly all the individual's emotional and social needs. Certainly the reality fails dramatically to live up to the image on the toothpaste adverts, for reasons that may be largely beyond the control of individual family members, although if we have succumbed to the 'happy families' myth we will be inclined to take the blame for such failings on ourselves alone, and even to insist and to believe that everything is fine in the face of over-whelming evidence to the contrary. Schizophrenic breakdown can be seen as one of the most dramatic challenges to this myth, although there are others too: as we have seen, the entangled patterns in families such as the Clarks differ in degree, not in kind, from families where the symptoms are less severe. For powerful protests like this, psychiatry reserves its most powerful treatment: the major tranquillizers.

At this point it is intriguing to note that the High EE (high expressed emotion) which is related to relapse in schizophrenia (Chapter 4) is a much less prominent feature of relatives in Chandigarh, North India, where there is an extended family structure, leading one writer to speculate that 'these Western responses to mentally disordered family members may be a product of emotional isolation engendered by nuclear-family life, or the result of high achievement expectations placed on the psychotic'.[8] This is fascinating research evidence of a link between the various levels that make up any psychiatric problem — the individual's personal experience, the marital/family context, and the political processes of the society in which they live.

A minority of other writers and mental health workers have also argued that individual distress can only be fully understood by placing it in a social/political context, and have pointed out the destructive consequences of a treatment approach that fails to take such factors into account. For example, Sheila Kitzinger, author of many books on pregnancy and childbrith, in writing about postnatal depression (though not about the more serious psychotic reactions which occasionally follow childbirth) is sceptical of the way that

> women are often told that postnatal depression is the result of a disturbed endocrine system and that it is all a matter of hormones. . . . It is only too easy to explain away and dismiss women's understandable frustration, anger, and despair about what life is doing to them by labelling it as 'premenstrual tension', 'menopausal neurosis', or 'postnatal depression'. . . . Many mothers feel somehow abandoned by society. . . . Most of us are not prepared for the resentment, the sense of inadequacy, guilt, anger, and murderous feelings we have as mothers. There is delighted discovery and joy and sometimes sheer ecstasy too, and that makes it all worthwhile. But the trouble is that the image of motherhood is romanticized. We learn nothing about how we are going to feel when woken by a crying baby for the tenth time between 3 a.m. and 5 a.m., or what it is like to be alone in the house with complete responsibility for a child for 8 to 10 hours a day. . . . Postnatal depression and despair is no accident, nor an act of God. It is the direct result of a society which puts motherhood on a pedestal while disparaging and degrading mothers in reality. . . . When a new mother becomes depressed or constantly anxious she is the victim of a social system which fails to value women as mothers and does not consider housework or child care real 'work', and in which she is cut off from the sources of self-esteem that all of us usually depend on and from the support which in traditional societies comes from other women in the extended family and neighbourhood. It is a social system which, when she cracks under stress, labels her as 'sick', offers her tranquillizers to keep her going instead of changing anything, and implicitly blames her for her failure to adjust. Postnatal depression and the distress which women experience when they become mothers is not their own private problem. It is a political issue, something which can only be changed when there is social change, and therefore a challenge to us all.[9]

And another example: a psychiatrist working with the elderly writes that although it is currently stated by practically all the textbooks that the aged are more prone to depression of an endogenous (i.e. without external cause) nature . . . we believe that the unhappiness which is misdiagnosed and mistreated as an endogenous illness is a legitimate response to the plight that many of the aged find themselves in. A number of studies have established that the aged are an oppressed group, they are poorer than the rest of the population, with 50 per cent of them on society's breadline, supplementary benefit. They have some of the worst housing and are eight times more likely to be isolated and alienated. Add to this the burden of physical disease and social prejudice and we have a social situation in which stress symptoms are inevitable. The so-called depression, therefore, is not primarily due to a biochemical upset but an understandable reaction to the alienation, rejection, isolation, and social stress that the aged are subject to. The diagnosis of depression has three dangerous aspects. First, it tells a person who is lonely, isolated, and poor that on top of it all, he is mentally ill. This, we believe, merely worsens his morale. Second, the diagnosis is associated with the prescribing of potent neuroleptics and sedatives which impair cognitive function and cause serious side effects. Finally it mystifies and medicalizes a problem, preventing its rational resolution. We believe that the treatment of so-called depression is to treat the causes of it. Poverty by the fuller use of available benefits, alienation by establishing relationships, and isolation by the use of caring networks, social clubs and day centres. Such 'treatments' may involve non-medical activity but it is preferable to prescribing pills which worsen the patient's confusion and serve mainly to swell the profits of powerful drug companies. [Using this approach, the team found that] the need for acute provision has been slashed to a fifth of the minimum laid down by the DHSS, more than 1,200 beds have been closed . . . we have the lowest drug bill in the country and none of our patients has committed suicide in over a decade.[10]

We have been looking at some of the social and political factors that form the background to individual distress and arguing that psychiatry, in so far as it ignores these factors and passes on the values and assumptions of the wider society with which it is identified, labelling dissent as illness, can be said to be performing the fundamental function of social control. If this is so, we should expect to find psychiatry reflecting and reinforcing other inbuilt prejudices of wider society as well. We have already discussed at some length how sexism in society is reflected in and reinforced by sexism in psychiatry at many different levels. The same is true for other forms of discrimination. Thus, although homosexuality is no longer officially categorized as a mental illness, gay men and women may still find that their sexual orientation is viewed as an abnormality and is seen as the cause of whatever other problems they may have. However, it is the effects of classism and racism in psychiatry that have been most thoroughly documented.

CLASSISM

It is well established that the working classes get a poorer deal than the middle classes in many areas. In 1980 the government tried to suppress the Black Report,[11] which attributed the greater risk of injury, sickness, and early death lower down the social scale to glaring inequalities in income, education, nutrition, housing, and working conditions. The 1987 report *The Health Divide*,[12] which updated these findings and confirmed that the gap between rich and poor had continued to widen, also met with attempts at suppression. As readers will have gathered from the stories presented in this book, working-class people are over-represented in the mental illness statistics as well. 'Numerous studies have revealed that there exists a strong association between social class and psychiatric disorder; that the highest rates of the latter are to be found in the lowest social groups.'[13] There are various possible explanations for this. One is that people with psychiatric problems tend to drift down the social scale as their ability to cope with more highly skilled jobs diminishes and lower salaries force them to move to cheaper neighbourhoods. Research studies disagree as to how much this does actually occur. Another possibility is that the greater stresses of a working-class environment actually contribute to the development of psychiatric problems in the first place. This is a difficult theory to test. As far as schizophrenia is concerned, it is considered to be unproven, though as one writer notes, it is rather perverse to acknowledge that increased life stresses in the lower classes can lead to higher rates of psychological symptoms, stress-related illness, and death, and yet make an exception for schizophrenia.[14] (Two American psychiatrists suggest that the discounting of social class factors in schizophrenia 'may . . . reflect the fact that influential research and clinical writing and teaching most often come from persons and institutions with predominantly upper- and middle-class orientations, while a large number of schizophrenic patients are lower class and unemployed'.)[15] A well-known study in Camberwell, London,[16] found that depression was much more common among working-class than among middle-class women, and that the stressful events experienced by the former were more numerous and more severe, typically lasting longer and being harder to resolve. Some examples were: husband being sent to prison, being threatened with eviction, being forced to have an unwanted abortion because of housing difficulties, and so on. Class differences were also relevant to some of the factors that made the women more vulnerable to depression in the first place, for example, having three or more children under fourteen at home, losing one's mother before the age of eleven, and the lack of a confiding relationship with someone, all of which are more typically features of working-class than of middle-class mothers. The whole issue is very complex and other factors are involved too. (Thus, for example, another study found that on the Isle of Wight as opposed to in London the association between social class and psychiatric disorder in women did not seem to hold.)[17] However, in general terms there is considerable evidence in support of a relationship between the particularly difficult social and economic circumstances of working-class life and consequently higher rates of psychiatric breakdown.

What is especially interesting from the point of view of the political role of psychiatry is the kind of treatment working-class people tend to receive. The staff hierarchy, descending from well paid, high status, middle-class doctors down through the ranks to working-class, low paid, low status domestics, reflects the whole structure of wider society. A number of studies have found that severer diagnoses are given to lower than to middle- class patients regardless of symptoms, that the former are seen as having a poorer prognosis, and that professionals are less interested in treating them. Working-class patients are more likely to be prescribed physical treatments such as drugs and ECT, to spend longer periods in hospital regardless of diagnosis, and to be readmitted, and correspondingly less likely to be referred for the more 'attractive' treatments such as psychotherapy and group therapy.[18] These referral patterns have been justified by the assertion that working-class patients are less articulate and therefore less able to benefit from verbal therapies, although this may simply reflect the difficulty that predominantly middle-class doctors and therapists have in understanding and communicating with people from very different cultural backgrounds and their inability to adapt their therapeutic approaches to take these differences into account. In any case, the end result is that those members of society who are least powerful and suffer most from social and economic hardship are most likely to receive the 'disabling' rather than the 'empowering' psychiatric treatments, which will tend to deprive them further of whatever degree of independence and autonomy they still retain. Again, the overall effect is to defuse legitimate protest, on an individual or a group level, by mystifying patients about the real origins of a substantial part of their difficulties.

RACISM

Similar themes have been traced in Littlewood's and Lipsedge's excellent book, *Aliens and Alienists*,[19] which looks at the experiences of ethnic minorities in psychiatry. Briefly, these two psychiatrists, while seeing mental distress as 'rooted both in biology and in culture, in the individual and in "society" ', argue that it can be an intelligible response to racism and disadvantage. Again, it is well established that these groups tend to do particularly badly in terms of housing, employment, and so on.[20] The authors found that 'the experiences of migration and of discrimination in housing, employment, and everyday life were frequently expressed by patients, not as conscious complaints, but symbolically in the actual structure of their illness'. For members of other cultures it is, or should be, especially obvious that what is 'normal' can only be judged in relation to their particular background, but unfortunately lack of appreciation of this fact has contributed to a situation where West Indian men are more likely to be admitted to psychiatric hospitals, psychotic black patients are twice as likely as British-born and white immigrants to be in hospital involuntarily, black patients are more likely to see a junior rather than a senior doctor, and even when differences in diagnosis are allowed for, black patients are more likely to be given major tranquillizers and ECT, while all minorities are less likely to be referred for psychotherapy.[21] Again, 'the dominant racialism in our society is reflected not just in the theories and practices of psychiatry but in its very structure: white consultants, Asian junior doctors, black nurses and domestics'.

The authors argue that 'the expression of mental illness, while it may not always be a valid communication to others, is still a meaningful reaction on the part of the individual to his situation', and a view of mental distress which ignores this aspect fits particularly badly in the case of ethnic minorities. For example, they present evidence to support their suggestion that the greater incidence of paranoid reactions among immigrants (believing that one is being spied on, that witchcraft is being practised against one and so on) may be 'merely a strong reiteration of the experience of discrimination'. Immigrant housewives who 'often experience such bad bodily pains, insomnia and bad dreams that they are unable to provide a secure domestic base for an ambitious husband to launch a career' can be seen as

protesting at their husbands' opportunities; he straddles two cultures, while for them life does not seem to have changed from that in their home country. While anger and frustration may occasionally be openly expressed, in the family they usually take the socially acceptable form of physical illness . . . the dominant political structure of the family can remain unthreatened.

They also discuss very interestingly how science and medicine have over the years been employed to 'prove' that members of ethnic minorities are different and inferior — that their brains are smaller (containing 'undifferentiated' and 'immature' nerve cells), that as childlike, happy savages in a state of nature they are incapable of experiencing depression, and more recently that blacks as a group have lower IQs than whites. The conclusions drawn are clearly in the interests of the dominant white section of society. (In America, for example, landowners were able to tell themselves that slaves who bolted were suffering from the mental illness of drapetomania — the irresistible urge to run away from plantations — rather than from dissatisfaction with the conditions under which they were forced to live and work.)

The authors argue the need for 'a psychotherapy that takes

into account the past and present relationship between European and non-European and which, while being sensitive to modes of expression such as religion, nevertheless does not regard minority mental illness as solely a "cultural problem" '. They conclude that 'consideration of normality and abnormality are not . . . "innocent" or value-free — we have seen that European attitudes to insanity in non-Europeans have been closely tied to political values', and more generally that 'the practice of psychiatry continually redefines and controls social reality for the community' — not just for ethnic minorities, but for us all.

The above illustrations of the social and political factors that form the background to individual distress have been little addressed in psychiatry, which is just what one would expect if its fundamental function of social control has to be concealed. It is not surprising then, to find that the relationship between the personal and the political has been most thoroughly explored *outside* psychiatry, although the book that links the whole field of mental health with a radical social critique in a thorough and convincing way has yet to be written. The failure to work out these theoretical issues contributed to the decline of the anti-psychiatry movement of the 1960s, personified by R. D. Laing, whose compelling books criticizing the medical view of mental distress had far more impact outside than inside psychiatry.

> Its vague theories, its detachment from traditional politics, and its disregard to strategy all seem to have condemned it — like flower-power — to wilt when the good vibes faded away. A much more hard-headed approach, both intellectually and politically, is required if the message of that movement is not to be completely lost today.[22]

One recent and impressive contribution to this task, coming, unusually, from within psychiatry itself, is psychiatrist Dr Richard Warner's book *Recovery from Schizophrenia*.[23] The remarkable achievement of Dr Warner is to have presented his very challenging conclusions in such a well-documented and scholarly way that he has drawn praise from highly respected mainstream psychiatrists such as Professor J. K. Wing. ('This is an intriguing book, full of ideas and surprises. Dr Warner is a scholar, well-versed in the huge international literature on schizophrenia. He juggles an immense array of biological, psychological, and social facts to create patterns that are always interesting and occasionally spectacular.')[24] The fact that Warner fundamentally adheres fairly closely to a medical model view of schizophrenia has undoubtedly contributed to this acceptance. For example, he appears to see no role for psychotherapy, either individual or family, beyond the problem-solving approach developed by Leff and his colleagues (Chapter 4). Nevertheless, the praise is well earned.

The argument of the book is complex and a summary cannot do it full justice. In essence, though, Warner is demonstrating the links between recovery rates from schizophrenia in different societies and the political economy of those societies, or, as he puts it in the introduction:

Does the way we make our living or the form of government under which we live affect whether or not we become insane? Does social class or the state of the economy influence whether schizophrenics recover from their illness? Has industrial development affected the number of schizophrenics who become permanently and severely disabled — lost to their families, costly to the country and leading lives of emptiness and degradation? These questions are at the heart of this book. . . . It is not only biological, genetic, or psychological factors which determine the distribution and course of schizophrenia. We should be prepared to expand our concern with social factors, beyond family dynamics and socioeconomic status. It is in the relationship between all of these potential causes and the economic, technological and environmental facts of our existence that we may gain the broadest understanding of why some people become schizophrenic and why some of them never recover.

Reviewing the research, Warner establishes, among other things, that fluctuations in the economy are associated with increased symptoms of psychological distress, that the stresses of both working and unemployment can create significant hazards to mental and physical health, and that mental hospital admissions for people of a working age increase during a slump — in other words, that there is a relationship between health, illness, and the economy.

He then turns to recovery rates from schizophrenia and demonstrates, with the help of sixty-eight studies from Europe and North America, that the prognosis (outcome) of this disorder has not in fact improved significantly since the beginning of the century, despite the claims attached to various treatment methods in turn — insulin coma, ECT, psychosurgery, and more recently the major tranquillizers. 'Despite the popular view in psychiatry, the anti-psychotic drugs have proved to be a critical factor in neither emptying mental hospitals nor achieving modern recovery rates in schizophrenia.'[25] In fact schizophrenia seems to have had the best prognosis of all in America during the era of moral treatment, the non-medical approach that emphasized a compassionate, respectful, and optimistic attitude to the mentally distressed (see Chapter 8), although American psychiatrists attempted to conceal this embarrassing fact by a dubious process of statistical juggling. Warner shows that what does correlate with recovery rates is the state of the economy, and more particularly the levels of unemployment — at times of high unemployment, prognosis is poorer, and vice versa. This sets the scene for him to argue that 'rather than psychiatric treatment having a big impact on schizophrenia, both the course of the illness and the development of psychiatry itself are governed by political economy.'

High unemployment can influence schizophrenia in various ways. Being unemployed is itself a stress, and Warner draws a telling comparison between the features of chronic schizophrenia:

> Patients may be abnormally tired, fatigue easily, and experience clinical depression. The chronic schizophrenic may sit blankly for long periods, unaware of the passage of time. . . . He may remain in bed when he intended to look for a job, avoid or put off without reason any activity that is new, unfamiliar or outside of his routine. . . . Life is routine, constricted, empty

and of long-term unemployment:

> cannot be bothered to do nowt, just feel like stopping in bed all day; I go for a walk and try to do some reading if I can, but it's very hard for me to get the brain functioning properly; I'm so *moody* you know; I think you start to lose your identity in yourself.

He notes that although 'in recent years . . . it has become so common for schizophrenics in the community to be out of work that mental health professionals rarely consider unemployment a significant stress for their patients', to label their deficits as biological rather than socially induced 'increases the pessimism regarding treatment and the stigma which attaches to the patient'. Warner also points out that

the similarity in the emotional reactions of the unemployed and of psychotic patients was highlighted by a study conducted in the Great Depression. The level of negativity and pessimism about the future in large samples of the Scottish and Lancashire unemployed was found to be greater than that of groups of psychotically depressed and schizophrenic patients. If the unemployed are as distressed as hospitalized psychotics, how can we hope that the unemployed psychotics will return to normal during hard times? In fact we may ask, as does the author of the study of the Scottish and Lancashire jobless, 'why the mentally distressed unemployed . . . do not become psychotic'. The answer is, of course, they may well do so. Brenner found that it was precisely that segment of the population which suffers the greatest relative economic loss during a depression — young and middle-aged males with moderate levels of education — which showed the greatest increase in rates of admission to New York mental hospitals for functional psychosis during an economic downturn.[26]

The other side of the picture is that periods of intense rehabilitation programmes and hence better prognosis — moral treatment, social psychiatry, and the 'Open Door' movement — were instituted in wartime or when there was a labour shortage. Moral treatment seems to have been particularly successful in America because there it was combined with a national demand for labour. Warner's argument — for which he advances a good deal of evidence — is that

the treatment of the great majority of the mentally ill will always reflect the condition of the poorest classes of society. . . . Despite the fact that an improvement in conditions of living and employment for psychotics may yield higher rates of recovery, this consideration will remain secondary. . . . Efforts to rehabilitate and reintegrate the chronically mentally ill will only be seen at times of extreme shortage of labour —

263

after the other battalions of the industrial reserve army have been mobilized. At other times, the primary emphasis will be one of social control.

During the latter times, psychiatry will tend to turn from an interest in the social causes of mental distress to an emphasis on biological and hereditary factors, with the sufferers being seen as untreatable. In other words:

> psychiatric ideology may be influenced by changes in the economy — a notion which implies a rejection of the conventional concept of scientific progress inherent in mainstream medical history. . . . Ideological views which emerge counter to the mainstream of psychiatric thought make no headway in the face of a contrary political and social consensus. . . . Ideology and practice in psychiatry, to a significant extent are at the mercy of material conditions.[27]

Warner then sets out to test various predictions that would follow from his argument. One is that the best outcome for schizophrenia will be found in the sex and social class that is least affected by labour market forces, and also in industrial nations with continuous full employment. And there is evidence in support of this: among women and the middle and upper classes, and in Switzerland (unemployment below 1 per cent since the Second World War) and the USSR (continuous full employment since 1930 and workers can expect jobs to be found for them even if they are barely productive) the prognosis is indeed better.

A further prediction is that outcome in schizophrenia will be better in non-industrial societies where wage labour and unemployment are uncommon. Turning to the Third World, Warner finds startling evidence against the assumption of western psychiatry that schizophrenia is a serious disorder that frequently leads to long-term disability. On the contrary, the more typical picture in the developing countries is of a brief episode with no lasting effects. Among various surveys pointing to this conclusion is a World Health Organization study of 1979 which used standardized methods of diagnosis and follow-up. Warner writes:

The general conclusion is unavoidable. Schizophrenia in the

Third World has a course and prognosis quite unlike the condition as we recognize it in the West. The progressive deterioration which Kraepelin considered central to his definition of the disease is a rare event in non-industrial societies, except perhaps under the dehumanizing restrictions of a traditional asylum. The majority of Third World schizophrenics achieve a favourable outcome. The more urbanized and industrialized the setting, the more malignant becomes the illness.[28]

This is despite the fact that in the Third World psychiatric care is often virtually non-existent, while in America up to 4 billion dollars a year is spent on the treatment of schizophrenia.

Warner advances a number of reasons for these extraordinary differences. One is that 'in non-industrial societies that are not based upon a wage economy, the term "unemployment" is meaningless'. Although *under*employment is common, it will be far easier for the individual to find some productive task which will make a contribution to the community and match his level of functioning at any given time. One would expect that in such societies, it would be the educated who suffer more acutely from labour-market stresses, and hence, in a reversal of the pattern in the developed world, have a worse outcome for schizophrenia, and Warner shows that this is so. And while peasant life is in many ways very hard, there are some features of it that are particularly favourable to the social integration of the mentally distressed. For example, symptoms such as hallucinations are far less likely to be labelled as madness, and the generally low level of stigma attached to mental disorder makes readjustment to family life much easier. Indeed, what we would call psychiatric symptoms can sometimes lead to an enhancement of social status. Moreover, the process of treatment in preindustrial societies is vigorous and optimistic, with the disorder more likely to be seen as a problem for the community as a whole, not just the individual. There is a strong emphasis on social reintegration — a factor that is closely related to outcome in all parts of the world. One especially interesting finding was the relationship between High EE (high expressed emotion) and the nuclear family structure mentioned earlier in the chapter.

Warner then turns to the question of whether political economy can actually trigger schizophrenia in the first place, as opposed to affecting the course of the condition once it has already developed. He marshals a complicated set of evidence to show, among other things, that schizophrenia is less common in the Third World than the west or in American communities like the Hutterites and the Amish where work and community support are assured; that migrant-labour practices may explain the increased risk of schizophrenia in some rural parts of the Third World; and that the Industrial Revolution in Britain may have caused a real increase in the occurrence of schizophrenia, quite apart from the other factors which led to overcrowding in the Victorian asylums. There are suggestions that insanity was much rarer in the non-industrial world before European contact and economic development.

Warner's depressing summary is this:

> Where pre-industrial cultures offer social integration with maintenance of social status and provision of a valued social role for many psychotics, Western society maintains schizophrenics in poverty and creates for them social disintegration with pariah status and a disabled role. In the non-industrial world, communal healing processes operate within a social consensus which predicts recovery and minimizes blame, guilt, and stigma; whereas in Western society schizophrenia is treated through marginal institutions with a social expectation that all concerned are to blame to a high degree and that the condition is incurable.

He believes that the situation of the western sufferer from schizophrenia is best summed up by Marx's concept of alienation, which is 'illustrated in the popular imagination by the assembly-line worker who is so disgusted and bored that he wilfully damages the car on which he is working'. It is the most dehumanizing and menial jobs that the psychotic patient is likely to find, but the fate of unemployment, which, Marx argued, is an unavoidable component of capitalist production, is even worse:

> To stand idle, to be unable to provide for oneself, to fulfil no useful social function, to be of no value to oneself or others — these are the ultimate in alienation . . . the origins of the schizophrenic's alienation are to be found in the political and economic structure of society — in the division of labor and the development of wage work.[29]

Following his lengthy analysis, Warner offers various suggestions for treatment. He sees a limited role for medication in some but certainly not all cases of schizophrenia (see Chapter 9), but believes that the most important ingredients will be 'stress reduction . . . close personal contact with staff and other residents . . . making appropriate plans for his or her life after discharge — finding a place to live and an occupation, neither of which should be too stressful', and so on. 'In short, aside from a lessened emphasis on stern paternalism and an increased emphasis on family relations, these treatment approaches attempt to recreate the principles of moral management as practised at the York Retreat.'[30] He believes that only a small number of patients are untreatable in the community, and that measures such as providing guaranteed jobs and training for the mentally disabled, a range of independent and supervised accommodation, support, and education for relatives, and so on would cost little more than the current vast social cost of treating and not treating schizophrenia as we do at present. His more general conclusion is less easy to implement. 'To render schizophrenia benign we may, in essence, have to re-structure western society.'[31]

The argument of Warner's book supports the contention that the primary function of psychiatry is not so much to treat (except where this happens to suit the political climate) as to maintain the status quo by absorbing and suppressing society's casualties and misfits, and labelling all their problems as illness. This, of course, is not something that can openly be admitted by psychiatry. Indeed to be seen to be acting politically, in the broadest sense, is to break one of the strongest taboos in psychiatric and psychotherapeutic circles. (In the narrower sense, political manoeuvring and power-games among the staff are endemic in the psychiatric system, as in other systems.) Psychiatrists strive to be scientific and objective, failing to realize that by, in effect, uncomplainingly sweeping up society's casualties and labelling their problems as illness they are already performing a very important political function — that in fact it is impossible *not* to act politically, and that to deny this is merely to add a layer of mystification to the process.

The same criticisms can be applied to the field of psychotherapy. Although this book has on the whole advocated psychotherapy as an alternative to physical treatments, it is important to remember that the former can be just as powerful a way of enforcing social norms as the latter, especially when practised by those therapists, who tend to be of a more psycho-analytic persuasion, who believe that they can conceal their own values and attitudes behind an interpretative, reflective, 'blank screen' approach. It has been pointed out that in America, where private, individual psychotherapy plays a much more important role than in Britain, the enormous growth of the mental health industry (most of the world's psychoanalysts, literally hundreds of new psychotherapies, self-help books of all kinds, and so on), can be said to be serving a very important political function at a time when, in the words of one critic, 'a special kind of mystification' is needed to conceal contradictions in the way the whole society is organized. 'It requires no feat of imagination to comprehend that capitalist society would come to reward the psychiatric profession for promoting a special type of psychological illusion', i.e. the illusion that the path to happiness and the answer to all problems lies in individual psychological exploration. 'The rise of a purely psychological view of human difficulties is a handy way of mystifying social reality.'[32]

Writers like Phyllis Chesler have pointed out how this applies in practice to women in particular:

For most women the middle-class oriented psychotherapeutic encounter is just one more instance of an unequal relation-ship, just one more opportunity to be rewarded for expressing distress and to be 'helped' by being (expertly) dominated. Both psychotherapy and white or middle-class marriage isolate women from each other; both emphasize individual rather than collective solutions to women's unhappiness. Each woman, as patient, thinks these symptoms are unique and are her own fault. She is neurotic rather than oppressed. She wants from a psychotherapist what she wants — and often cannot get — from a husband: attention, understanding, merciful relief, a *personal solution* — in the arms of the right husband, on the couch of the right therapist. . . . This is probably not a coincidence but is rather an expression of the American economic system's need for geographic and psycho-logical mobility, i.e. for young, upwardly mobile 'couples' to 'survive', and to remain more or less intact in a succession of alien and anonymous locations, while they carry out the functions of socializing children and making money. Most therapists have a vested interest, financially and psychologically, in the supremacy of the nuclear family.[33]

Behaviour therapy, which again has made particular claims to be scientific and objective, has sometimes been for this very reason equally guilty of covertly promoting particular norms and values. Before homosexuality was legalized between consenting adults, male homosexuals were routinely offered aversion therapy — administering electric shocks at the same time as showing them sexually arousing pictures of men — as an alternative to prison, with the first option being described as 'treatment' rather than punishment. The behavioural programmes of shopping and cooking that are offered to depressed housewives have already been described. During the vogue for what are known as token economy systems, whole wards of patients had their behaviour regulated by depriving them of cigarettes and other treats unless they dressed and acted in ways deemed acceptable by the staff.

And it is not only Warner who has pointed out the circular process whereby psychiatric theories are influenced by cultural beliefs, and then used to justify and give 'scientific validity' to whatever is politically expedient. Penfold and Walker, two Canadian mental health workers, describe how the work of Bowlby and others on the supposedly devastating effects of mother-infant separation and maternal deprivation was both influenced by traditional assumptions (fathers are virtually unmentioned) and then used by legislators to justify not providing child-care facilities and keeping mothers out of the workforce. More generally, they argue that

psychiatric theories that blame mothers and their families allow society to avoid looking at and trying to alleviate the numerous pressures that families face today, including poverty, unemployment, discrimination, poor housing, lack of stable support systems, unsuitable educational programmes, and a variety of emotional stresses. . . . We have to take a new look at whether our theories about mother-infant attachment, child development, and family relationships are valid and scientific or whether they merely reflect cultural beliefs and thus serve both to perpetuate the status quo in our society and to hide the fact that the social structures themselves may be at fault.[34]

Perhaps the only instance of a treatment philosophy which openly admitted the values on which it was based was moral treatment. Although, as was pointed out in Chapter 8, this approach reinforced social norms just as firmly as more punitive regimes — patients were expected to conform to a strict code of moral behaviour, behave themselves nicely at specially arranged tea-parties and so on — since there was no attempt to conceal the aims of cure, the patients were at least clear about the rules of the game. Currently there are very few examples of approaches which are equally transparent, one exception being the feminist psychoanalytic approach developed by Orbach and Eichenbaum at the Women's Therapy Centre in London.

We have already seen from Warner's analysis how innovations are only permitted to flourish at all if the political climate favours it; reforms 'make no headway in the face of a contrary political and social consensus'.[35] In a related process, reforms that are implemented with genuinely benevolent intent tend to be absorbed into the system where they eventually come to serve the same purpose of upholding the prevailing order. An example was the Mental Hygiene Movement in America, founded in 1908 on the impetus of an ex-patient's account of the horrific conditions in mental asylums. By the First World War, it had become involved in government projects for the psychological health of the forces; and moreover it has been argued that the whole concept of 'Mental Hygiene' contributed to the development of a positivist model for separating off the unhygienic, insanitary aspects of mental life and labelling deviance as sickness in need of an expert cure.[36] The more radical the innovation, the greater is the need to reinterpret it by stripping it of its revolutionary aspects and harnessing its power to the establishment. This is what has happened to Christianity: adopted as the official religion of the Roman Empire in AD 312 it has a long history of use by the state to justify repressive policies. Transactional Analysis, originally a therapy with a very radical component, is widely used in sanitized versions to train executives and salespeople to clinch deals and maximize profits. It has been argued that Freud and psychoanalysis are victims of the same phenomenon.[37] The danger is that the community care movement will fall a victim to the same process, that it will turn out to be nothing more than a means of exporting social control and the medical model to a wider audience in the community.

We are all familiar with the idea that in some countries

psychiatry is overtly used to suppress those who are critical of the political system, or 'those who think differently', the literal meaning of the Soviet term for dissidents. Without necessarily suggesting that British and western psychiatry is guilty of just as much abuse as the Soviet version, it can be argued that there is a difference of degree, not of kind, between the two systems. Consider, for example, these two accounts of the experience of being on psychiatric drugs:

I have been given two tablets of [the drug] twice daily, that is four tablets in all, and [the chief psychiatrist] assures me that this will go on for a long time. This medicine makes me feel more awful than anything I have experienced before; you no sooner take a step than you're longing to sit down, and if you sit down you want to walk again — and there is nowhere to walk.[38]

After ten days or so, the effects of [the drug] began building up in my system and my body started going through pure hell. It's very hard to describe the effects of this drug and others like it, that's why we use strange words like 'zombie'. But in my case the experience became sheer torture. Different muscles began twitching. My mouth was like very dry cotton no matter how much water I drank. My tongue became all swollen up. My entire body felt like it was being twisted up in contortions inside by some unseen wringer.[39]

Which is the Soviet dissident being punished in order to make him recant his criticisms of society, and which is the mentally ill westerner receiving psychiatry's most effective treatment for psychosis? The drugs are the same — the major tranquillizers. The dividing line between treatment and torture can be a very narrow one. (The first is a Russian hunger striker in a special hospital, and the second a young American.)

In the USSR as in the west, the smokescreen behind which the function of social control can be carried out is the use of the medical model. The veil is rather thinner in the USSR which employs such concepts as 'sluggish schizophrenia', an interesting variation of the condition in which the usual delusions and hallucinations are absent — indeed there may be 'no clear symptoms' at all, although Soviet psychiatrists have argued that one should not be misled by the 'seeming normality of such sick persons when they commit socially dangerous actions'.[40] Soviet citizens are apparently also liable to sinister syndromes such as 'paranoid delusions of reforming society' and 'hippieism'. However, we have seen that the superficially more rigorous and respectable use of the medical model in the west in fact conceals an equal number of implicit social judgements and ultimately serves the same function of social control, although in a country where it is more important to maintain the myth of democracy and freedom of thought, both staff and patients and the general public may need to be more profoundly mystified about the whole process.

As David Ingleby has pointed out,[41] the medical model which provides such a useful vehicle for this process of social control is itself only one example of positivism — the particular way of thinking that underlies nearly all scientific research and enquiry and is also deeply rooted in the minds of ordinary people. The scientist, according to this model, is someone who collects observation in an objective and detached manner, eliminating all traces of subjectivity and bias, testing and discarding theories in order to come to an ever more complete knowledge of the laws of nature. By adopting this approach from the natural sciences, psychiatry has tried to give itself an air of respectability and impartiality. (Psychology has tried to do the same by its claim to be rooted in the scientific and proven principles of behaviourism, largely based on experiments on laboratory animals, or as Ingleby caustically puts it, 'has sought to apply to human problems a theory which barely fits the albino rat'.)[42] Not everyone has been convinced by this manoeuvre: 'Psychiatry is a subject with very poor experimental substantiation for its claims of aetiology and treatment. . . . Medical students . . . see it as a mess, as a complete muddle in which they can certainly find no way through',[43] as one young doctor explained the widespread aversion of his peers to the speciality. Moreover, as we have seen, there are rather serious shortcomings to the positivist, medical approach of 'studying human beings as if they were things' — the inability to define basic psychiatric terms, the existence of bias in diagnoses, the absence of evidence for physical causation, the damage inflicted by psychiatric treatments, the failure to produce significant rates of cure, and most fundamentally, the loss of the person and of personal meaning. However, rather as the predictable debunking of particular psychiatric treatments fails to lead to a questioning of the whole rationale for using physical treatments in psychiatry at all, the objections outlined above have only led to an increasingly urgent desire to shore up the illusion with scientific research, to the point where 'the literature on mental disorders is quite out of proportion to the adequacy of our knowledge about them.'[44] The reams that have been written on diagnosis are an important example. To admit to the existence of the extra 'unscientific' factors that contribute to a diagnostic label (except by glossing over the problem with talk of the small amout of 'clinical judgement' that is involved) would be to give the whole game away, because if there is no agreement on basic classification, then the field of psychiatry can never be developed into a science. 'Diagnosis is the Holy Grail of psychiatry and the key to its legitimation.'[45]

Another manoeuvre of the increasingly sophisticated medical model is to disarm its critics by assimilating aspects of different approaches without actually changing its basic, positivist standpoint. Thus we saw in Chapter 8 how nineteenth-century doctors, threated by the success of moral treatment, adopted some of its ideas themselves and then claimed that only they, as the people who understood both medical and non-medical approaches, were qualified to be in charge of the whole enterprise. What this did was to reduce moral treatment from a whole philosophy of care to a mere collection of techniques. Psychotherapy has met a similar fate; while more enlightened psychiatrists agree that it has a part to play and may even practise psychotherapy themselves, this psychotherapeutic understanding is an addition to, not a replacement for, the basic medical model one. Similarly, what is known as 'social psychiatry' does acknowledge the importance of social factors — but, in accordance with a respectable, scientific approach, is only willing to address them by divesting them of their meaning. Social factors become just another variable to be added into the formula — inadequate personality plus marital disharmony plus redundancy equals reactive depression, and so on. What it actually *means* to a man to be unemployed after twenty years in work, what it actually *feels like* to be a woman bringing up three children in a high-rise flat on a restricted income — such matters cannot be discussed within a positivist medical model framework. In this way, the connection between life as subjectively experienced by the individual and the conditions of the wider society of which she or he is a part is disguised. The individual is

273

seen not so much as an active social agent as an object to be tuned and adjusted by experts. Such an approach is in marked contrast to feminist analyses of women's psychology which have drawn out the links between external social and political conditions (women's restricted position in society, the different roles they are expected to fulfil etc.) and the personal, internal psychological experience of individual women themselves (low self-esteem, over-investment in emotional relationships, and so on).

The notion that there can be such a thing as objective, value-free scientific research and practice has in fact been challenged from within science itself. It has also been argued, by critics like Elizabeth Fee, that the generally accepted assumption that the positivist, scientific, objective, detached, abstract approach is in some way intrinsically better, truer, more valid than any other can be seen as just another example of the predominance of masculine values in contemporary society. As she puts it, 'We find that the attributes of science are the attributes of males. . . . Science is cold, hard, impersonal, "objective"; women, by contrast, are warm, soft, emotional, "subjective". . . . We can expect a sexist society to develop a sexist science.'[46] She argues, as Ingleby and others have argued of medical model psychiatry, that this so-called objectivity and the concept of the pursuit of knowledge for its own sake as an abstract and value-free ideal, is a myth which allows the covert promotion of particular political interests. Fee suggests that a science which incorporated traditionally female values as an essential and equally valid aspect of human experience would reduce the gap between the production of knowledge and its uses which sanctions 'the political passivity of those scientists who have tacitly agreed to accept a privileged social position and freedom of inquiry within the laboratory in return for . . . not questioning the social uses of science'. It would challenge the separation of thought and feeling which 'may be employed to devalue any positions expressed with emotional intensity or conviction; feeling becomes inherently suspect, the mark of an inferior form of consciousness' — an attitude that leads to the curious sterile language of scientific journals. It would change the one-way flow of information from scientific expert to non-experts who, lacking official credentials, are made to feel uninformed and unintelligent and unable to contribute to debate. In short, such a science would readmit the human subject, and 'seek to integrate all aspects of human experience into our understanding of the natural world'.

Such an approach as applied to psychiatry would challenge medical model attitudes whereby the individual person and his/ her feelings are virtually eliminated from view and psychiatrists attain eminence not by learning to understand and relate to their patients as people but by adding to the mountain of academic research; where the commonsense intuitions of ordinary people (such as the comments of clerical staff in Chapter 7) are ignored in favour of abstract theorizing which bewilders laypeople and junior members of staff with its impression of lofty expertise; and where the personal experiences of patients are discounted (thus, the 'widespread conviction by former patients that their memories have been permanently affected' by ECT was abruptly dismissed in a review article, Chapter 9) by quoting research and statistics. It would also rehabilitate one notable casualty of the psychiatric system, psychotherapy, which emphasizes traditionally feminine qualities such as intuition and emotional expression. Most importantly of all, a science which incorporated traditionally female values would challenge the medical model notion that the practice of psychiatry can be apolitical and value-free. As Warner has argued, psychiatric ideology and the development of psychiatry itself 'may be influenced by changes in the economy — a notion which implies a rejection of the conventional concept of scientific progress inherent in mainstream medical history'.

Medical model psychiatry is, of course, only the most recent in a long line of measures which various societies have employed to deal with their deviant members, although there is a natural tendency to believe that contemporary viewpoints are 'the truth', as magical and religious explanations were regarded in their time. It is in fact no more 'true' to say that mental distress is caused by biochemical abnormalities than by witchcraft or by a Mafia conspiracy to poison your tea, although the latter type of explanation, sometimes put forward by patients diagnosed as paranoid, may have a personal meaning which at least provides a starting point for some kind of human understanding of the problem. The time is long overdue for a new metaphor, a new way of understanding mental distress, and the overthrow of the whole medical model tradition. This, according to a writer who has studied the evolution of scientific ideas, is

what scientists never do when confronted by even severe and

prolonged anomalies. Though they may begin to lose faith and then to consider alternatives, they do not renounce the paradigm (i.e. the whole pattern of thinking) that has led them into crisis. They do not, that is, treat anomalies as counter instances. . . . They will devise numerous articulations and ad hoc modifications of their theory in order to eliminate any apparent conflict.[47]

The crucial hidden function of social control provides the impetus for this frantic shoring up of the model. However, as one critic has said, 'If history has any predictive validity at all, we can assume that our current ideas in this area are transitory and will eventually meet the same fate as their predecessors.'[48] Let us hope that this is so.

In the meantime we can draw together, in the last chapter, some tentative suggestions for change.

12

Pointers to the future

A good place to start is by acknowledging that not all aspects of the present psychiatric system are unhelpful or harmful. There are skilful and dedicated members of staff, and there are patients who benefit from their contact with psychiatry. Medication and admission are useful to some people as part of the help they need. The old Victorian asylums with their extensive grounds can be an ideal retreat for the severely disturbed in the acute stage of their distress. Medical training is essential to detect the small minority of problems that have their origin in clearly physical causes.

However, all is not right, and the faults are embedded at a very fundamental level of the system. Former users of the service are in the best position to comment on the results:

> The tedium of the evenings oppressed almost everyone, and the boredom at the weekends afflicted those who did not take weekend leave. We all felt we were very much in the power of the hospital authorities. Although we were free to discharge ourselves at any time, few were in a condition to do so, and so long as one stayed in hospital, one had to agree to the conditions imposed. . . . None of us liked the constant surveillance, and many of us felt oppressed because we could not deal on equal terms with nurses or doctors; we were mad; they did not need to take us seriously.

> My own view is that the staff were too kind; I think this contributed very greatly to the 'infantilization' I instantly recognized among my fellow-patients, who were not made to

lift a finger to help themselves. . . . Everyone was doped to the eyeballs. Most just went to the dayroom for meals (when they felt like it) and drifted back to lie on their beds between meals.

The nurse took my tablets off me and made a final brisk squiggle on her clipboard. 'There's a list of mealtimes and a washing-up rota on the noticeboard upstairs', she said. 'Toilets and bathroom down to the corridor on the left. If you want a bath ask the nurse for the taps.' It was as simple as that. Ten minutes ago I had been a responsible adult. Now I was a patient in a psychiatric unit and had to ask for the bath taps.

One of the worst periods in hospital is when you're well and you can't convince anyone you're well. Somehow you have got to sell your sanity to the nurses and the doctor and it is very easy to fluff it.[1]

Some former users of the psychiatric services are banding together and demanding to be heard, for instance, members of the collective who made a Channel 4 TV programme[2] on their experiences in hospital:

I got involved with the programme because I felt that psychiatry was about suppressing symptoms. So-called 'symptoms' are isolated and assessed out of context with a person's internal and external environments or their political, sociological, emotional, or physical pressures. The psychiatric institution sits as prosecuting barrister, judge, jury, jailer, and in some cases executioner. The defendant (the 'troubled' person) is assumed to be perjuring themselves and the only verdicts are guilty in varying degrees. In helping make the programme, I have had a chance to express, with others, the overwhelming anger, frustration, revulsion, and horror that I feel, in a way that is more accessible than the voiceless impotence of being on the receiving end of psychiatry. . . . When I was being treated by psychiatry I felt that I had little or no say in my own life. It was assumed that I was unable to make decisions. I had a label that invalidated me in the eyes of the community and thus in my own eyes too. The criteria for the stigma are learnt very young. (I have heard school children say I was mad and should be locked up.) My perception of my environment was said to be faulty. I was given drugs that inhibit perception.

Another user said:

I became involved in making this film fifteen years after my six-month brush with the psychiatric system. It had taken me ten years to put my life back together and to begin to understand how psychiatry had damaged and confused me. My contact with other ex-patients and making this film has helped me realize that I have a right to be angry because however much individuals within the psychiatric system may care about their patients, the system as a whole works to control and silence people, not enable them to grow and learn and live through their crisis and pain. I am the best judge of my own experience. I do not need psychiatry's labels and diagnosis to tell me what I feel. The way psychiatry invalidates its victims and dispossesses them of their human rights has a long history; 'scientific knowledge' and 'clinical judgement' are only the most recent justifications. In the past, the church or the state were the authorities which demanded conformity, and would kill, lock up, or re-indoctrinate those who rebelled. . . . Psychiatry dramatically reinforced the passive role, which, as a working-class woman, I had already been trained for, but which I had been trying to reject. It has taken me long years since to regain my confidence — years which I believe psychiatry has robbed me of. My crisis could have been a positive turning point in my life, from which I gained the strength to redefine myself. This is what we should be fighting for — a new understanding of crisis — not as illness, but as opportunity — and a psychiatric system which serves and respects those in pain, distress, and trauma, instead of controlling and exploiting them.[3]

The determination of former users to organize and protest is vital if anything is to change. This involves giving up what for many people is a very deep-rooted desire to find an expert with a magic answer and a magic pill to put them right, and taking power into their own hands instead. After all, if patients are no longer willing to play at being patients, psychiatric staff can no longer play at medical model psychiatry.

My own proposals are pointers rather than blueprints for a

perfect system. In the same way that mental distress needs to be understood at a number of different levels, change needs to occur at many different levels as well.

First, there is the level of the help that is given to individuals in mental distress. Examples of how this needs to change have been given throughout the book. To recapitulate briefly, mental distress needs to be understood not as an illness to be treated by medical means (which is the message that traditional psychiatric treatment conveys, either explicitly or implicitly by falling back on the medical approach in default of alternatives), but as something that has to do with the *whole person* and all of their past and present experiences, existing in a *whole system* of relationships. Psychotherapy, whether individual, marital, family, or group, needs to be available to everyone who can benefit from it, even if in the end the most appropriate intervention is behaviour therapy, simple rest and relaxation, social support, or whatever — or no intervention at all. This therapeutic understanding should not start and end during scheduled sessions, but should be applied to all of a person's experience and behaviour while they are being cared for. It should equally be extended to relatives, who besides needing support and full information about what is being done to help the person in need, may benefit from psychotherapeutic help themselves.

Equally important is attention to the person's *social circumstances* — their housing, finances, social contacts, local sources of support, job situation, and so on — and a commitment to offering practical rather than medical help where social factors play an important part in the problem. In addition to the information already possessed by social workers, this would mean all members of staff knowing about local organizations and resources — housing associations, advice bureaux, job training schemes, day centres, hostels, clubs, crèches, and so on — and seeing it as part of the service's function to set up projects such as home help for mothers who are in temporary need during a crisis, and support groups and social clubs for the isolated, all these to be located in non-medical settings that are part of the local community and used for a variety of non-psychiatric purposes to avoid the implication of illness and the segregation that is usually imposed on the mentally distressed. Familiarity with the catchment area — its housing, transport, shops — is essential for all staff.

As we saw in earlier chapters, it is not only the kind of help that is offered, but the way it is offered that is so important. In order to avoid entrance into the sick role and the whole destructive Rescue Game, where patients typically progress from 'mad' to 'bad' collecting all sorts of derogatory labels on the way, the use of *treatment contracts* must be standard. This means that the patient (and the relatives if they are to be involved too) has made an explicit request for help with a clearly defined problem; that an equally explicit offer of a clearly described and understood form of help has been offered; that the person understands the contribution she or he will be expected to make to this form of help; and that she or he has accepted the offer. (This includes the right to refuse any help at all.) Clear contracts are especially important where treatments that carry an 'illness' message — drugs, admission — are involved, and needless to say should include full information about risks and side effects. These treatments should never be the only help given, but if offered and accepted as outlined above may be a useful adjunct to other forms of help. We saw in Chapter 4 how the treatment contract approach can be applied in the case of severely distressed individuals. The underlying assumption, in contrast to the medical model view, is that people in mental distress are fundamentally *equal and responsible human beings*, even if currently in need of extra support.

The help that is offered must be directed towards *empowering* rather than disabling the person in distress. On the whole this will mean an emphasis on the less readily available options such as counselling and psychotherapy and support in the community, rather than the standard medical routine of drugs and admission. It should also imply a view of mental distress as a potentially positive experience, an *opportunity for growth and change* if the clues can be deciphered, rather than an unfortunate episode that needs to be defused and suppressed as quickly as possible. A commitment to empowering will also involve greater recognition of the fact that although trained staff do have particular skills to offer, people who are or have been in mental distress themselves can give each other unique and valuable help, support, and understanding. Group therapy makes the most powerful use of these assets (although it so happens that most of the examples in this book are of individual therapy). Women's groups, men's groups, mixed groups, ward groups, and self-help and support groups of all types can be set up with the explicit aim of utilizing the insight, experience, and care of ordinary people.

Extending these principles up to the next level would obviously involve fundamental changes in the way mental health staff are trained, so that *training is based on a psychotherapeutic and social understanding of mental distress* and not, as is still the case with psychiatrists, nurses, and occupational therapists, on the modified principles of general medicine. The situation where most mental health professionals acquire psychotherapeutic skills, if at all, as a kind of optional extra after the official training is quite untenable — as is the lack of training in counselling for GPs who deal with most of the psychiatric problems in the general population, and are the gateway to psychiatric treatment. The widespread ignorance of the range of therapies that have been developed, mostly in America, over the last forty years is equally regrettable. Art Therapy and Music Therapy are slowly gaining a place for themselves. There have been glimpses of two personal favourites, Transactional Analysis and Gestalt, earlier in this book. Others that are well worth investigating, although there is no space to describe them here, are Psychodrama and Dramatherapy, in which clients explore their problems by role-playing them; Bioenergetics and one of its offshoots, Postural Integration, which have broken the mould of traditional psychotherapy by working with and through the body; Neuro-Linguistic Programming, which has distilled powerful therapeutic techniques from the close study of various outstanding therapists; Co-counselling, which emphasizes an egalitarian, non-professional relationship in which each person takes it in turn to be counsellor and client; and many others. Although individual members of staff and different professions may retain and develop their own expertise and interests, the destructive consequences of the divided-function approach to mental distress could be avoided by rooting all skills in a broader psychotherapeutic framework, which might form a core professional training, where the care and understanding of the whole person is seen as everyone's role and responsibility. Equally importantly, staff support groups and therapy groups should be a standard part of training and of jobs, so that the carers are cared for themselves, and the personal change and development that is necessary if patients are also to change and develop can occur.

Training also needs to promote *awareness of sexism, classism and racism* (and of discrimination on the grounds of age, sexual orientation, and so on). There should be an active commitment to ensuring that these conditions are not reflected and reinforced in psychiatry, so that, for example, black staff have an equal chance of achieving positions of responsibility, or the traditionally female tasks such as cooking are not taught exclusively by female staff. Entrance requirements may need to be adapted to encourage a broader cross-section of people to apply for training. Psychotherapy often has a particularly middle-class orientation. Several researchers have drawn attention to the need for psychotherapy to be adapted to take into account the different experiences, expectations, and needs of ethnic minorities and working-class clients, traditionally seen as poor therapeutic prospects. Various attempts to do this, by, for example, preparing both therapists and clients in advance, being willing to adopt a more flexible, commonsense attitude focusing on practical issues and giving advice where necessary, avoiding jargon and so on, show that it is possible to avoid high drop-out rates and achieve good results.[4]

These suggestions have implications for the whole way the service is organised. *Crisis intervention* (a cohesive team making a thorough assessment of all potential admissions in the home setting) with a crisis intervention philosophy (seeing crisis as a unique opportunity for therapy and change) is the best way to avoid the setting up of the treatment barrier, the Rescue Game and its consequences. Moreover, if all staff are to play a genuinely equal (though not necessarily identical) role in admission and treatment, the whole hierarchy needs to be reorganized along democratic lines. Although medical expertise has its place, there is no good reason why doctors should automatically head the psychiatric team. In some community-based services, for example, referrals are made to the whole team, which may be headed by a member of any profession or may have a rotating chairperson, and are shared out among staff each of whom has their own independent caseload. In a proper community care programme staff will find themselves crossing traditional professional boundaries, and in fact MIND has argued for the creation of a new profession, the community mental health worker, whose role incorporates aspects of the nurse, psychologist, occupational therapist, and social worker. The logical extension of democratization and shared responsibility would be equal pay scales for all mental health professionals.

Power should not only be redistributed down the staff

hierarchy; *power must be extended to users of the service* as well. The logical extension of viewing them as equal and responsible agents who play an active part in the treatment process is to involve them equally in the way the whole service is run. This means not only giving open access to medical files and to staff discussions about patients and routinely asking for consumer feedback on the service, but also having patient representatives on management boards and interview panels and staff training programmes. There are a few places where this has started to happen. Nottingham has a system of Patient Councils in wards, days centres, and community mental health centres, which aim to promote the interests of users and ex-users of the service. They are involved in staff appointments and are running a drop-in centre. In Holland all psychiatric hospitals have Inmates' Councils, organized at a national level with three government-funded workers, which must by law be consulted on certain subjects such as the building of new wards or the introduction of new treatments. A willingness to utilize the experience of ex-patients by employing them as therapists in their own right would be one of the most effective ways of breaking down the us versus them, sick versus healthy barrier, although it would also be very threatening to the status of the professionals. Advocacy schemes, whereby people outside the service can be used to represent the needs and interests of users, can give a mouthpiece to those who find it difficult to speak up for themselves.

Many of the ideals outlined above — sharing of responsibility, decision-making by consensus, blurring of roles, flattening of the authority pyramid, freeing up communication, using the therapeutic skills of patients — were embodied in the therapeutic community movement that had its heyday in the 1950s. Only when these are fully put into practice can the users of the psychiatric services legitimately be called clients rather than patients.

Psychiatry as a whole needs to make *closer links not only with social services but with the many voluntary and self-help organizations* that do so much to fill the gap left by the official services, and it needs to be willing to use, support, and learn from them. Operating from a non-medical point of view, these organizations have developed expertise in areas as varied as rape, incest, violence, abortion, marital and sexual problems, eating problems, bereavement, alcoholism, and many others. They also have considerable experience in setting up and running hostels, night shelters, halfway houses, and other facilities.

At present psychiatry's main focus is on treating acute distress, with a lesser but increasing emphasis on rehabilitation of those who are more disabled. *Preventative work* is virtually non-existent, and it has been argued that more time should be devoted towards education for mental health — for example, running courses on child-rearing, preparing for retirement, dealing with stress — although possibly this kind of function falls more appropriately to the education system. Moving towards community care implies a greater involvement with the community as a whole — its businesses, churches, trade unions, schools, its festivals and public events — in order to reverse the pariah status that psychiatry and psychiatric patients have traditionally been assigned.

Research in psychiatry needs to turn away from the medically respectable refining of diagnostic categories and quest for obscure physiological correlates of mental distress which have so little practical application, and *readmit the whole person and his/her personal experience and relationships* as a legitimate focus of study. Needless to say, funding from sources other than drug companies needs to be made available for this purpose. If categorization and classification is to be used in psychiatry, then the absence of reliability and validity of the present medical model system must first be acknowledged, and more meaningful constructs which do not eliminate the person and the social and relationship system within which she or he lives must be developed instead. While the academic papers pile up, the areas in which research is genuinely needed — unbiased investigation of the risks of psychiatric treatments, consumer surveys of psychiatric care, the connection between mental distress and social and political factors, theoretical models that link the personal with the political — are virtually ignored.

The next level up is local and central government. MIND's manifesto, *A Better Life*,[5] based on

> the belief that the experience of mental illness should not be a barrier to the enjoyment of the full rights and responsibilities of citizenship. The right to a home, to food, to an adequate income, to employment, to self-determination, to choice and to participation in the social, cultural and political life of a community is the same for a person with mental illness as for every other citizen

285

has a ten-point charter of necessary steps for the community care policy:

At least another £500 million a year to meet real, desperate needs for mental health services.

A central bridging fund to make possible the transition from hospital to community care.

A comprehensive disability income and costs allowance, paid as of right, which takes into account the added costs imposed by mental illness.

The restoration of the 50 per cent cut in the Housing Investment Programme and the provision of ordinary and supported housing in the community.

A comprehensive, non means-tested carers' benefit.

Retraining and redeployment for staff currently working in institutions and a policy of no compulsory redundancies.

A public education programme to combat the stigma and prejudice against mental illness.

Planning together for community care with health authorities, local government, service users, and the voluntary sector collaborating on plans for new local services. A team of government ministers must start working jointly on national policies.

Giving greater and more detailed attention to mental health issues and policies both in Parliament and in national and local political debate.

Listening to the views of people who have used mental health services — the true voices of experience.

MIND has particularly emphasized the crippling effects of poverty on mental health. For the 17 million people who depend on the state for their main source of income, trying to make ends meet is a constant stress; the difficulty of doing so is a major feature in the lives of people admitted to psychiatric hospitals and a handicap in their attempts to rebuild their lives in the community.

Warner has put forward similar recommendations: providing guaranteed jobs and training for the mentally disabled which is neither too demeaning nor too stressful; ensuring adequate psychological and clinical support in the community, including a full range of independent and supervised, non-institutional accommodation; providing adequate material support, including an income which allows a decent status and standard of living;[6] and so on.

Reforms of the drug industry, which plays such a crucial role in psychiatry, are long overdue. Generic substitution (in which pharmacists would automatically dispense the cheaper generic version of a drug unless the doctor specifically indicated to the contrary) would be a useful start. One investigator has proposed a number of ways in which corporate crime in the drug industry could be controlled[7] — for example, by setting up independent drug regulatory bodies and consumer groups with legal standing and power, having a probation period for the limited marketing of new drugs and a mechanism for immediate withdrawal if problems emerged, and various other measures. The fact that drastic reforms are possible is shown by the experience of Bangladesh, where, despite intense opposition from the industry and from other interested parties, a recommended list of generic drugs for the Government's health system was drawn up, one-third of the country's medicines were thrown out, and strict price controls were introduced, with the result that prices have fallen while quality has improved.

Moving onto a wider level, the *general public needs to take responsibility for becoming aware and informed about mental health issues*. There are several good reasons for this. One is that by doing so they can understand better what happens to friends and relatives who receive psychiatric treatment, and can avoid becoming victims of the psychiatric system themselves. Another is so that they can press for the reforms that seem unlikely to come from within the system itself. The third and perhaps most important reason is that psychiatry and psychiatric staff are only performing the function that we, members of the general public, overtly or covertly demand of them; thus, we are all intimately involved in the abuses of the system. One of the most dangerous myths of our age is that we as individuals are not involved in the crimes that go on around us. In fact we are all involved — in the arms race, in pollution, in Third World hunger — although our involvement generally takes the form of sins of unawareness and of omission, or of small actions that have a cumulative effect. As society becomes more complex, our involvement becomes not only more indirect but also more mystified — thus, the control of deviance is often dressed up as help rather than punishment. If the psychiatric system is to change, each one of us needs to be more tolerant of dissidence or 'thinking differently' in other people, to be willing to befriend, employ, and live near or with sufferers from mental distress, and to take back into ourselves some of the confusion, fear, and despair that at the moment (like men who leave their wives to carry all the feelings in the marriage, or families who locate all the craziness in one member) we require psychiatric patients to bear on behalf of all of us. We need to listen to the messages that the lives of those who have fallen to the bottom rung of society carry for us and our whole way of life.

Ultimately we need to *move away from, and eventually abandon altogether, the whole medical model approach* which, this book has argued, underlies all the other flaws in psychiatry. This means screening out and separating off those problems with a clearly physical origin (where disturbance can be traced to head injury, senile dementia, brain tumours, and so on) which can legitimately be seen as needing medical care in addition to other kinds of support and advice. Non-medical places of refuge, where 'asylum' in the original sense of the word can be obtained, should be available for those who desperately need a break from their personal circumstances. In some places the community care policy is to move away from hospitals altogether and instead set up a number of small local crisis units in ordinary houses adapted for the purpose. Most of the medical knowledge that is useful in helping the mentally distressed, for example, advising on whether a tranquillizer might have a part to play and what the possible side-effects are, could be included as part of the training that all mental health professionals receive, rather than being the exclusive province of doctors. In fact, reversing the nineteenth-century alignment of psychiatry with general medicine would mean that although the mental health team will need to have access to a doctor for treatment of any physical illnesses and conditions from which patients may incidentally be suffering, or that may be compounding their psychological difficulties, the medical profession has no essential part to play in helping the mentally distressed at all. It would also mean, as Foudraine (Chapter 10) found in his reforms, that we need a whole new vocabulary that gets away from the medical connotations of terms like hospital, patient, ward, nurse, treatment, and illness, and that describes the experience of mental distress in straightforward, jargon-free terms that everyone can use and understand.

The thread that runs through all these reforms must be *political awareness* — a conscious realization that the problem of mental distress and how to deal with it is at the most basic level a political one. Without this awareness, all the reforms in the world will not really change anything — and may even make the situation worse. We have already seen in Chapter 11 how innovations tend to flourish only when the political climate favours them, and how reforms that are implemented with genuinely benevolent intent tend to get absorbed into the existing system. We have also seen that psychotherapy can be just as powerful a way of covertly enforcing social norms as physical treatments. What is needed, then, at all levels of the help that is offered to the mentally distressed, is a philosophy and an approach that is *aware of its own values and assumptions*, makes them *explicit to the client*, *offers the client a choice* as to whether or not she or he agrees with or wishes to act on these values and assumptions, and *makes the necessary support available* if the answer is yes. It is vital that the final choice be left to the client, or else such an approach will be just as guilty of imposing its values on the client as the traditional one; and it is equally vital to start from where the client stands at present, rather than prescribing a plan for revolutionary action which may be as unwelcome and inappropriate as a prescription for tranquillizers. In summary, since there is no such thing as an objective, value-free approach to mental distress, the aim would be at the very least to demystify the client about the values held by the therapist and implicit in the treatment. The aim of the therapist then becomes, in the words of one of them, 'to help reveal the meaning of experience, to "demystify" it by liberating it from the normalizing ideology of our time . . . One sides with the person rather than the social world, helping to drag out his or her *internalized* norms so that they can be seen for what they are: the *external* disciplinary apparatus of a fundamentally oppressive social organization. At the very least, this gives people the freedom to think and feel what they like, to examine their experience for its significance rather than simply for its "abnormality".' It would then be up to the client to decide whether he or she agreed with this approach and wanted to take things further, and whether to translate the inward struggle into an outward one.

The full implications of such a philosophy remain to be worked out, and, if adopted, imply a continual process of questioning and discussion and re-evaluation of attitudes and beliefs on the part of the staff, rather than the attainment of some absolute level of awareness. Translated into practical terms, such an approach would not necessarily look very different. There is no occasion or time for a political polemic when an acutely distressed person is in urgent need of help, and equally, most simple phobias do not merit a lengthy analysis on the state of society. In other cases the differences would probably seem minor, although they may be crucial. For a therapist working with a depressed housewife, for example, it would be necessary not only to refrain from prescribing cooking-and-shopping programmes, but also to avoid saying, directly or indirectly, 'What you need to do is drop all the housework/get a job/leave your husband' and so on, statements which carry an equally powerful message about the way she should be. Instead, discussion might start with the therapist making his or her position explicit: 'It is my belief that a woman has a right to a life of her own apart from her family obligations. Do you agree? What implications would that have for you in your situation? Do you want to try and put that belief into practice? Where do you want to start? How far do you want to take it? What help do you want from me along the way?' The woman now knows what assumptions this therapy will be based on, and has a choice whether or not to continue with it. She also has a choice as to how and how far to translate these values into her own life — and her own personal revolution, the way in which she chooses to challenge her own mini-system, may consist of something as small as allowing herself a cup of coffee during a shopping trip, or taking an hour off to have an undisturbed bath, or buying herself a magazine from the housekeeping money (actual examples from clients). In these seemingly insignificant ways, individuals who wish to do so can be supported and encouraged to translate wider political movements (for example, the woman's movement) into their own personal lives. But whether or not such strategies are relevant in an individual case, an awareness of the broader political implications of one's actions and interventions must form the background to all the work that mental health professionals undertake. At a higher level this will mean mental health workers seeing it as part of their job to take an active role in lobbying and campaigning, preparing reports and putting pressure on official bodies, not necessarily on party political grounds, but on issues such as transport, housing, poverty, and unemployment if these are believed to play an important part in leading to mental distress and breakdown; and to support and encourage users of the service in doing the same. And at the most general level, the existence of mental distress poses very fundamental questions for all of us about our whole aggressive, competitive, achievement-oriented society in which traditionally feminine values are so heavily outweighed by traditionally masculine ones.

None of these reforms will happen overnight, and nor should they, if the internal process of becoming aware of our values and assumptions and our identification with the present system is to keep pace with the external signs of change. With systems as with individuals, change has to start from where people actually are and adapt itself to their pace, and it has to start not from a position of blame, but with everyone taking responsibility for their own contribution. If individuals can change — which they can — then systems can do so too. The necessary first step in any real change is creating awareness. I hope this book will be a contribution to that process.

Notes

CHAPTER 1

1. Department of Health and Social Security (1986) *Health and Personal Social Services Statistics for England.* HMSO.
2. *Health and Personal Social Services Statistics*, op. cit.

CHAPTER 2

1. Swarte, J. in H. Freeman (ed.) (1969) *Progress in Mental Health.* London: Tavistock.
2. Tring, J. L. (1970) 'The hierarchy of preference towards disability groups', *Journal of Special Education* 4: 295–306.
3. This diagram is adapted from S. B. Karpman (1968) 'Script drama analysis', *Transactional Analysis Bulletin* 7, 26: 39–43.

CHAPTER 3

1. Parsons, T. (1951) 'Illness and the role of the physician: a sociological perspective', *American Journal of Orthopsychiatry* 21: 452–60.
2. Ullmann, L. P. and Krasner, L. (1975) *A Psychological Approach to Abnormal Behaviour*, 2nd Edition, p. 354. New York: Prentice-Hall Inc.
3. This description of treatment contracts is derived from C. Steiner (1975) *Scripts People Live*, pp. 290–99. New York: Bantam Books.

CHAPTER 4

1. Hirsch, S. R. and Leff, J. P. (1975) *Abnormalities in Parents of Schizophrenics.* Maudsley Monograph no. 22. London: Oxford University Press.
2. Gelder, M., Gath, D., and Mayou, R. (1983) *Oxford Textbook of Psychiatry*, p. 259. Oxford: Oxford Medical Publications.
3. Grad, J. and Sainsbury, P. (1968) 'The effects that patients have on their families in a community care and a control psychiatric service: a 2-year follow-up', *British Journal of Psychiatry* 114: 265.
4. For example, see D. Ingleby in D. Ingleby (ed.) (1981) *Critical Psychiatry: The Politics of Mental Health.* Harmondsworth: Penguin.
5. Warner, R. (1985) *Recovery from Schizophrenia: Psychiatry and Political Economy*, p. 26. London: Routledge & Kegan Paul.
6. Heston, L. L. (1966) 'Psychiatric disorders in foster-home-reared

children of schizophrenic mothers', *British Journal of Psychiatry* 112: 819–25.

7. Foudraine, J. (1974) *Not Made of Wood: A Psychiatrist Discovers his own Profession*, p. 365. London: Quartet Books.

8. Vaughn, C. E. and Leff, J. P. (1976) 'The influence of family and social factors on the course of psychiatric illness: A comparison of schizophrenic and depressed neurotic patients', *British Journal of Psychiatry* 129: 125–37; Leff, J. P. and Vaughn, C. E. (1981) 'The role of maintenance therapy and relatives' expressed emotion in relapse of schizophrenia: A two year follow-up', *British Journal of Psychiatry* 139: 102–4; Leff, J., Kuipers, L., Berkowitz, R., Eberlein-Vries, R., and Sturgeon, D. (1982) 'A controlled trial of social intervention in the families of schizophrenic patients', *British Journal of Psychiatry* 141: 121–34.

9. Brown, G. W. and Wing, J. K. (1972) 'Influence of family life on the course of schizophrenic disorders: a replication', *British Journal of Psychiatry* 121: 241–58.

10. Leff *et al.* (1982), op. cit.

11. Berkowitz, R. (1984) 'Therapeutic intervention with schizophrenic patients and their families: a description of a clinical research project', *Journal of Family Therapy* 6: 211–33.

12. Leff *et al.* (1982), op. cit.

13. Sturgeon, D., Turpin, G., Kuipers, L., Berkowitz, R., and Leff, J. (1984) 'Psycho-physiological responses of schizophrenic patients to high and low expressed emotion relatives: A follow-up study', *British Journal of Psychiatry* 145: 62–9.

14. Scott, R. D. (1973a) 'The treatment barrier: Part 1', *British Journal of Medical Psychology* 46: 45–55.

15. Scott, R. D. (1975) ' "Closure" in family relationships and the first official diagnosis'. Paper presented at the Fifth International Symposium on the Psychotherapy of Schizophrenia, Oslo.

16. Scott, R. D. (1973a), op. cit.

17. Scott, R. D. (1975), op. cit.

18. Scott, R. D. (1973b) 'The treatment barrier: Part 2, The patient as an unrecognized agent', *British Journal of Medical Psychology* 46: 57–67.

19. Scott, R. D. (1973b), op. cit.

20. Scott, R. D. (1973a), op. cit.

21. Scott, R. D. (1960) 'A family-oriented psychiatric service to the London Borough of Barnet', *Health Trends*, 12: 65–8.

22. 'Crisis in mind', *Nursing Times* 22 July 1976.

23. Scott, R. D. and Seccombe, P. (1976) 'Community psychiatry — setting up a service on a shoe-string', *Mindout* 17, July/August: 5–7.

24. Ratna, L. (1978) 'Crisis intervention and community care, a comparative study', in *The Practice of Psychiatric Crisis Intervention*. Published by The League of Friends, Napsbury Hospital.

25. Langsley, D. *et al.* (1968) *The Treatment of Families in Crisis*. New York: Grune & Stratton; Decker, J. and Stubblebine, M. (1972) 'Crisis intervention and prevention of psychiatric disability: a follow-up

study', *American Journal of Psychiatry* 129 (6): 710.

26. Schiff, J. L. (1975) *Cathexis Reader: Transactional Analysis Treatment of Psychosis*, p. 3. New York: Harper & Row,
See also: Schiff, J. L. and Day, B. (1970) *All My Children*. Philadelphia: J. L. Lippincott Co.

27. Schiff, *Cathexis Reader*, op. cit., p. 99.

28. Schiff, J. L. (1977) 'One hundred children generate a lot of TA', in G. Barnes (ed.) *Transactional Analysis after Eric Berne*. New York: Harper & Row.

CHAPTER 5

1. Department of Health and Social Security (1986) *Health and Personal Social Services Statistics for England*. London: HMSO.

2. Bart, P. B. (1971) 'Depression in middle-aged women', in V. Gornick and B. K. Moran (eds) *Women in Sexist Society: Studies in Power and Powerlessness*. New York: Basic Books.

3. Eichenbaum, L. and Orbach, S. (1983) *Outside In, Inside Out: Women's Psychology: A Feminist Psychoanalytic Approach*. Harmondsworth: Pelican.

4. Eichenbaum and Orbach (1983), op. cit., p. 35.

5. Orbach, S. (1986) *Hunger Strike*. London: Faber & Faber.
Chernin, K. (1983) *Womansize: The Tyranny of Slenderness*. London: Women's Press.

6. Wardle, J. and Beales, S. (1986) 'Restraint, body image, and food attitudes in children from 12–18 years', *Appetite* 7: 209–17.

7. Report in the *Independent*, 1988.

8. Calloway, P., Fonagy, P., and Wakeling, A. (1983) 'Autonomic arousal in eating disorders: further evidence for the clinical subdivision of anorexia nervosa', *British Journal of Psychiatry* 142: 38–42.
Bhanji, S. and Mattingly, D. (1981) 'Anorexia nervosa: some observations on "dieters" and "vomiters", cholesterol and carotene', *British Journal of Psychiatry* 139: 238–41.

9. MIND Special Report, *Minor Tranquillisers: Hard Facts, Hard Choices*. MIND Publications.

10. Woodward, S. and Lacey, R. (1985) *That's Life! Survey on Tranquillizers*, pp. 27–8. British Broadcasting Corporation in association with MIND.

11. Brown, G. W. and Harris, T. (1978) *The Social Origins of Depression*. London: Tavistock.

12. Broverman, I. K., Broverman, D. M., Clarkson, F. E., Rosenkrantz, P. S., and Vogel, S. R. (1970) 'Sex-role stereotypes and clinical judgements of mental health', *Journal of Consulting and Clinical Psychology* 34: 1–7.

13. For example, C. R. Brown and M. Hellinger (1975) 'Therapists' attitudes towards women', *Social Work* 20: 266–70.

14. Abramowitz, S. F., Abramowitz, C. V., Jackson, C., and Gomes, B. (1973) 'The politics of clinical judgement: What non-liberal examiners infer about women who do not stifle themselves', *Journal*

of Consulting and Clinical Psychology 41: 385–91.

15. Starr, I. (1985) 'The depressed sex?', *Social Work Today*, 26 August.

CHAPTER 6

1. *About Men*, TV programme.
2. Ingham, M. (1985) *Men: The Male Myth Exposed*, pp. 7–8. London: Century Publishing.
3. Ingham, M. (1985), op. cit., pp. 10, 14.
4. Rubin, L. (1985) *Intimate Strangers*. London. Fontana/Collins. This account of men's psychological development is largely derived from Ms Rubin's book.
5. Moss, H. (1976) 'Sex, age, and state as determinants of mother-infant interaction', *Merrill-Palmer Quarterly* 13: 19–36.
6. Penfold, P. S. and Walker, G. A. (1983) *Women and the Psychiatric Paradox*, p. 103. London: Eden Press.
7. Penfold, P. S. and Walker, G. A. (1983), op. cit., p. 104.
8. Furman and Markman, (details not known).
9. Feinblatt, J. A. and Gold, A. R. (1976) 'Sex roles and the psychiatric referral process', *Sex Roles* 2 (2): 109–21.
10. Rubin, L. (1985), op. cit.
11. Starr, I. (1985) 'The depressed sex?', *Social Work Today*, 26 August.
12. Dohrenwend, B. P. and Dohrenwend, B. S. (1976) 'Sex differences and psychiatric disorders', *American Journal of Sociology* 81 (6).
13. Warr, P. (1983) 'Work, jobs and unemployment', abbreviated version of paper presented to the British Psychological Society, April 1983.
14. Warner, R. (1985) *Recovery from Schizophrenia: Psychiatry and Political Economy*, p. 52. London: Routledge & Kegan Paul.
15. Brenner, M. H. (1973) *Mental Illness and the Economy*. Cambridge, Mass.: Harvard University Press.
16. Warr, (1983), op. cit.
17. Warr, (1983), op. cit.
18. Hodson, P. (1984) *Men: An Investigation into the Emotional Male*, pp. 15, 95, 93. London: British Broadcasting Corporation, BBC Publications.
19. Dr Robert Sharpe quoted in P. Hodson (1984), op. cit., p. 101.
20. Kinnersley, P. (1973) *The Hazards of Work: How to Fight Them*. London: Pluto Press.
21. American Psychiatric Association (1980) *Diagnostic and Statistical Manual III*, 3rd Edition. Washington DC: APA.
22. Hill, D. (1985) *The Politics of Schizophrenia*, p. 204. London: University Press of America.

CHAPTER 7

1. Farrell, B. A. (1973) 'The place of psychodynamics in psychiatry', *British Journal of Psychiatry* 143: 1–7.
2. Littlewood, R. and Lipsedge, M. (1982) *Aliens and Alienists: Ethnic Minorities and Psychiatry*, p. 21. Harmondsworth: Penguin.
3. 'Who puts medical students off psychiatry?', p. 7. A meeting of the Association of Psychiatrists in Training held at the London Hospital Medical College on 6 February 1979, published by Smith, Kline, and French Laboratories Ltd.
4. Littlewood, R. and Lipsedge, M. (1982), op. cit., p. 21.
5. 'Who puts medical students off psychiatry?', pp. 22, 23.
6. Clare, A. (1980) *Psychiatry in Dissent: Controversial Issues in Thought and Practice*, 2nd Edition, p. 402. London: Tavistock.
7. Perinpanayagam, quoted in Clare (1980), op. cit., p. 403.
8. Shepherd, M., Cooper, B., Brown, A. C., and Kalton, G. W. (1966) *Psychiatric Illness in General Practice*. London: Oxford University Press.

CHAPTER 8

1. *Henderson and Gillespie's Textbook of Psychiatry* (1969), 10th Edition, p. 1. London: Oxford University Press.
2. Scull, A. T. (1979) *Museums of Madness: The Social Organization of Insanity in Nineteenth-Century England*, p. 15. Harmondsworth: Penguin.
3. Clark, W. *Remarks on the Construction of Public Hospitals for the Cure of Mental Derangement*, quoted in Scull, op. cit., p. 134.
4. Nesse Hill, G. *An Essay on the Prevention and Cure of Insanity*, quoted in Scull, op. cit., p. 135.
5. Nisbet, W. *Two letters to . . . George Rose MP on the Reports at present before the House of Commons on the State of Madhouses*, quoted in Scull, op. cit., p. 135.
6. Higgins, G. *The Evidence taken before a Committee of the House of Commons respecting the Asylum at York; with observations and notes*, quoted in Scull, op. cit., p. 140.
7. Ellis, W. *Letter to Thomas Thompson MP*, quoted in Scull, op. cit., p. 140.
8. Higgins, quoted in Scull, op. cit., p. 140.
9. Tuke, S. *Description of the Retreat*, quoted in Scull, op. cit., p. 143.
10. *Journal of Mental Science*, quoted in Scull, op. cit., p. 165.
11. Tuke, D. H. *History of the Insane*, quoted in Scull, op. cit., p. 170.
12. Kraepelin, E. (1962) *One Hundred Years of Psychiatry*. London: Peter Owen.
13. Granville, J. M. *The Care and Cure of the Insane*, quoted in Scull, op. cit., p. 195.
14. Ackner, B., Harris, A., and Oldham, A. J. (1957) 'Insulin

treatment of schizophrenia — a controlled study', *Lancet* 2: 607–11.

15. Hunter, R. and Macalpine, I. (eds) (1963) *Three Hundred Years of Psychiatry*. Oxford: Oxford University Press.

16. Quoted in W. Freeman (1968) *The Psychiatrists*, pp. 47–8. New York: Grune & Stratton.

17. Tooth, G. C. and Newton, M. P., quoted in A. Clare (1980) *Psychiatry in Dissent; Controversial Issues in Thought and Practice*, 2nd Edition, p. 283. London: Tavistock.

18. Robin, A. and MacDonald, D. (1975) *Lessons of Leucotomy*. London: Henry Kimpton.

19. Scull, A. (1984) *Decarceration: Community Treatment and the Deviant, A Radical View*, p. 80. Cambridge: Polity Press.

20. Hill, D. (1986) 'Tardive Dyskinesia: a worldwide epidemic of irreversible brain damage', in N. Eisenberg and D. Glasgow (eds) (1986) *Current Issues in Clinical Psychology*. Aldershot: Gower.

21. Scull, A. (1984), op. cit., p. 82.
Warner, R. (1985) *Revovery from Schizophrenia: Psychiatry and Political Economy*, p. 72. London: Routledge & Kegan Paul.
Treacher, A. and Baruch, G. (1978) *Psychiatry Observed*, p. 52. London: Routledge & Kegan Paul.

22. MIND Special Report: *Anti-Depressants, First choice or last resort?* MIND publications.

23. Cade, J. F. J. (1949) 'Lithium salts in the treatment of psychotic excitement', *The Medical Journal of Australia* 3 September: 349–52.

24. Warner, R. (1985), op cit., p. 19.

25. Hughes, R. and Brewin, R. *The Tranquillizing of America*, p. 36. New York: Harcourt Brace Jovanovich.

26. Hughes, R. and Brewin, R., op. cit., p. 193.

27. Lacey, R. and Woodward, S. (1985) *That's Life! Survey on Tranquillizers*. British Broadcasting Corporation in association with MIND.

28. Hunt, quoted in Scull (1984), op. cit., p. 96.

29. Powell, J. E. (1961) Address to National Association for Mental Health Annual Conference.

30. World Health Organization (1953) *Expert Committee on Mental Health — Third Report*, quoted in A. Treacher and G. Baruch (1978), op. cit., p. 81.

31. US Department of Health and Human Services (1981) *Toward a National Plan for the Chronically Mentally Ill*, Part 2, p. 11. Department of Health and Human Services Publication Number (ADM) 81–1077.

32. *Inpatient Statistics from the Mental Health Enquiry for England 1982*, HMSO, Department of Health and Social Security, first published 1985.

33. Warner, R. (1985), op. cit., pp. 121–5.

34. Clare, A. (1980), op. cit., p. 55.

CHAPTER 9

1. Braithwaite, J. (1984) *Corporate Crime in the Pharmaceutical*

Industry, p. 159. London: Routledge & Kegan Paul.

2. Klass, A. (1975) *There's Gold in Them Thar Pills*, p. 72. London: Penguin.

3. Hughes, R. and Brewin, R. *The Tranquillizing of America*, p. 9. New York and London: Harcourt Brace Jovanovich.

4. Lacey, R. and Woodward, S. (1985) *That's Life! Survey on Tranqillizers*, p. 25. BBC in association with MIND.

5. Blackwell, B. (1977) *The Sociopharmacology of Minor Tranquillizers*. Presentation to World Congress on Mental Health, Vancouver.

6. Hill, D. (1986) 'Tardive dyskinesia: a worldwide epidemic of irreversible brain damage', in N. Eisenberg and D. Glasgow (eds) *Current Issues in Clinical Psychology*. Aldershot: Gower.

7. Lacey, R. and Woodward, S. (1985), op. cit., p. 44.

8. Tiranti, D. (1986) 'A pill for every ill', *The New Internationalist* 165, November.

9. Braithwaite, J. (1984), op. cit., pp. 172–6.

10. Medawar, C. (1984) *The Wrong Kind of Medicine?* Consumer's Association and Hodder & Stoughton.

11. Braithwaite, J. (1984), op. cit., p. 165.

12. Medawar, C. (1984), op. cit., p. 6.

13. Melville, A. and Johnson, C. (1982) *Cured to Death: the Effects of Prescription Drugs*, p. 68. London: Secker & Warburg.

14. Braithwaite, J. (1984), op. cit., p. 215.

15. Braithwaite, J. (1984), op. cit., p. 214.

16. Penfold, S. P. and Walker, G. A. (1983) *Women and the Psychiatric Paradox*, p. 199. Montreal and London: Eden Press.

17. Medawar, C. (1984), op. cit., p. 37.

18. Penfold, S. P. and Walker, G. A. (1983), op. cit., p. 198.

19. Melville, A. and Johnson, C. (1982), op. cit., p. 51.

20. Tiranti, D. (1986), op. cit.

21. Braithwaite, J. (1986) 'The corrupt industry', *The New Internationalist* 165, November.

22. Braithwaite, J. (1984), op. cit., p. 259.

23. Braithwaite, J. (1984), op. cit., p. 265.

24. Braithwaite, J. (1984), op. cit., p. 34.

25. Medawar, C. (1984), op. cit., p. 48.

26. Braithwaite, J. (1984), op. cit., p. 310.

27. Braithwaite, J. (1984), op. cit., p. 2.

28. Braithwaite, J. (1986), op. cit., p. 20.

29. Medawar, C. (1984), op. cit., p. 59.

30. Association of the British Pharmaceutical Industry, quoted in C. Medawar, (1984), op. cit., p. 62.

31. Medawar, C. (1984), op. cit., p. 44.

32. Medawar, C. (1984), op. cit., p. 66.

33. Tyrer, P. (1979) 'The basis of drug treatment in psychiatry', in P. Hill, R. Murray, and A. Thorley *Essentials of Postgraduate Psychiatry*, p. 628. London: Academic Press.

34. Greenblatt, D. J. and Shader, R. I. (1980) 'Meprobamate: a study of irrational drug use', quoted in P. Schrag (1980) *Mind Control*. London: Marion Boyars.

35. Schrag, P. (1980), op. cit., p. 112.

36. Schrag, P. (1980), op. cit., p. 142.

37. Peck, R. E. 'The miracle of shock treatment', quoted in P. R. Breggin (1979) *Electroshock: Its Brain-Disabling Effects*, p. 9. New York: Springer.

38. Silverman, M. and Lee, P. R. (1974) *Pills, Profits and Politics*, p. 82. Berkeley: University of California Press.

39. Lacey, R. and Woodward, S. (1985), op. cit., p. 23.

40. Lacey, R. and Woodward, S. (1985), op. cit., p. 58.

41. Lacey, R. and Woodward, S. (1985), op. cit., p. 60.

42. Lacey, R. and Woodward, S. (1985), op. cit., p. 58.

43. *The Independent*, Tuesday 24 February, 1987.

44. Lacey, R. and Woodward, S. (1985), op. cit., p. 63.

45. Lacey, R. and Woodward, S. (1985), op. cit., p. 35.

46. The Committee on the Safety of Medicines, in *Journal of the Medical Defence Union*, Summer 1988.

47. *The Observer*, 20 March 1988.

48. Warner, R. (1985) *Recovery from Schizophrenia: Psychiatry and Political Economy*, p. 239. London: Routledge & Kegan Paul.

49. Breggin, P. R. (1983) *Psychiatric Drugs: Hazards to the Brain*, p. 35. New York: Springer.

50. 'Living with schizophrenia' in *Mind's Eye*, published by Channel 4 Television, September 1986.

51. Baldessarini, R. J. and Lipinski, J. F. 'Toxicity and side-effects of antipsychotic, antimanic and antidepressant medication', quoted in D. Hill (1986), op. cit., p. 95.

52. Hill, D. (1986) op. cit., p. 91.

53. Fann, W. E., Smith, R. C., Davis, J. M. and Domino, E. F. (eds) 'Tardive dyskinesia: research and treatment', quoted in D. Hill (1986), op. cit., p. 95.

54. MIND Special Report, *Major Tranquillizers — The Price of Tranquillity*. MIND Publications.

55. Hill, D. (1986), op. cit., p. 90.

56. Hill, D. (1986), op. cit., p. 94.

57. Breggin, P. R. (1983), op. cit., p. 109.

58. Warner, R. (1985), op. cit., p. 259.

59. Warner, R. (1985), op. cit., p. 143.

60. Warner, R. (1985), op. cit., pp. 242–4.

61. Warner, R. (1985), op. cit., p. 246.

62. Rappaport, M., Hopkins, H. K., Hall, K. *et al*. 'Are there schizophrenics for whom drugs may be unnecessary or contraindicated?' quoted in R. Warner (1985), op. cit., p. 250.

63. Breggin, P. R. (1983), op. cit.

64. Breggin, P. R. (1983), op. cit., pp. 126–40.

65. Grant, I., Adams, K. M., Carlin, A. S., Rennick, P. M., Judd L. L., and Schoof, K. 'The collaborative neuro-psychological study of polydrug users', quoted in P. R. Breggin (1983), op. cit., p. 139.

66. MIND Special Report, op. cit.

67. MIND Special Report, op. cit.

68. The Royal College of Psychiatrists (1977) 'Memorandum on the

use of electroconvulsive therapy', *British Journal of Psychiatry* 131: 262–72.

69. *Henderson and Gillespie's Textbook of Psychiatry* (1969) revised by I. Batchelor, Tenth Edition, p. 326. London: Oxford University Press.

70. Kendell, R. E. (1981) 'The present status of electroconvulsive therapy', *British Journal of Psychiatry* 139: 265–83.

71. The Royal College of Psychiatrists (1977), op. cit.

72. Pippard, J. and Ellam, L. (1981) 'Electroconvulsive treatment in Great Britain', *British Journal of Psychiatry* 139: 563–8.

73. Breggin, P. R. (1979) *Electroshock: Its Brain-Disabling Effects.* New York: Springer.

74. Pippard, J. and Ellam, L. (1981), op. cit.

75. Breggin, P. R. (1979), op. cit., p. 36.

76. Breggin, P. R. (1979), op. cit., p. 36.

77. Kennedy, A. 'Critical review of the treatment of mental disorders by induced convulsions', quoted in P. R. Breggin (1979), op. cit., p. 141.

78. Group for the Advancement of Psychiatry, Report no. 1: *Shock Therapy*, quoted in P. R. Breggin (1979), op. cit., p. 145.

79. Hartelius, H. 'Cerebral changes following electrically induced convulsions', quoted in P. R. Breggin (1979), op. cit.

80. Kalinowsky, L. and Hoch, P. 'Somatic treatments in psychiatry', quoted in Breggin, *Electroshock*, op. cit.

81. Karl Pribram quoted in Breggin, *Electroshock*, op. cit., p. 145.

82. R. J. Grimm quoted in Breggin, *Electroshock*, op. cit., p. 123.

83. Jones, J. E. (1974) 'Non-ECT', *World Medicine* September: 24.

84. Kendell, R. E. (1981), op. cit.

85. Johnstone, E. C., Deakin, J. F. W., Lawler, P., Frith, C. D., Stevens, M., McPherson, K., and Crow, T. J. (1980) 'The Northwick Park ECT trial', *Lancet* ii: 1317–20.

86. MIND Special Report, *ECT: Pros, Cons and Consequences*, Mind Publications.

87. Clare, A. (1980) *Psychiatry in Dissent: Controversial Issues in Thought and Practice*, 2nd Edition, p. 266. London: Tavistock Publications.

88. MIND Special Report, *Anti-Depressants. First Choice or Last Resort?* Mind Publications.

89. Meredith, T. J. and Vale, J. A. 'Poisoning due to psychotropic agents'.

90. *Anti-Depressants. First Choice or Last Resort?* op. cit.

91. Schou, M. (1986) 'Lithium treatment: a refresher course', *British Journal of Psychiatry* 149: 541–7.

92. National Institute of Mental Health booklet quoted in Breggin, *Psychiatry Drugs*, op. cit., p. 187.

93. Mander, A. J. (1986) 'Is there a lithium withdrawal syndrome?' *British Journal of Psychiatry* 149: 498–501.

94. Edwards, S. and Kumar, V. (1984) 'A survey of prescribing and psychotropic drugs in a Birmingham psychiatric hospital', *British Journal of Psychiatry* 145: 502–7.

95. Michel, K. and Kolakowska, T. (1981) 'A survey of prescribing psychotropic drugs in two psychiatric hospitals', *British Journal of Psychiatry* 138: 217–22.

96. Clark, A. F. and Holden, N. L. (1987) 'The persistence of prescribing habits: a survey and follow-up of prescribing to chronic hospital inpatients', *British Journal of Psychiatry* 150: 88–91.

97. Edwards, S. and Kumar, V. (1984), op. cit.

98. Michel, K. and Kolakowska, T. (1981), op. cit.

99. Jus et al., quoted in Hill, D. (1986), op. cit., p. 98.

100. Royal College of Psychiatrists' report, 1981, quoted in *ECT: Pros, Cons and Consequences*, op. cit.

101. Boulter, A. and Campbell, M. 'An ethnography of minor tranquillizer use in selected women's groups in Vancouver', quoted in Penfold, S. P. and Walker, G. A. (1983), op. cit., p. 191.

102. *Major Tranquillisers — The Price of Tranquillity*, op. cit.

103. *Anti-depressants: First Choice or Last Resort?* op. cit.

104. *Major Tranquillisers — The Price of Tranquillity*, op. cit.

105. Kendell (1981) op. cit.

106. Pippard and Ellam (1981) op. cit.

107. *Major Tranquillisers — The Price of Tranquillity*, op. cit.

108. Warner, op. cit., p. 258.

109. Dr Malcolm Peet interviewed in *Asylum* 1 (2) Summer 1986.

110. Tiranti, D. (1986), op. cit.

111. Lacey, R. and Woodward, S. (1985), op. cit., p. 45.

112. Braithwaite, J. (1984), op. cit., p. 204.

113. Gorring quoted in Braithwaite, *Corporate Crime*, op. cit., p. 205.

114. Unpublished figures from the Home Office in *Drug Link*, July/August 1986, vol. 1, issue 2.

115. Warner, R. (1985), op. cit., p. 164.

116. Braithwaite, J. (1984), op. cit., p. 344.

117. Tyrer, P. (1979), op. cit., p. 628.

118. Ingleby (1981) Understanding 'Mental Illness', in D. Ingleby (ed.) *Critical Psychiatry: The Politics of Mental Health*, p. 37. Harmondsworth: Penguin.

CHAPTER 10

1. Kurt Lewin quoted in Introduction to J. Foudraine (1974) *Not Made of Wood: A Psychiatrist Discovers his own Profession*. London: Macmillan.

2. Foudraine, J. (1974), op. cit.

3. Foudraine, J. (1974), op. cit., pp. 3–4.

4. Foudraine, J. (1974), op. cit., Introduction.

5. Foudraine, J. (1974), op. cit., Introduction.

6. Foudraine, J. (1974), op. cit., pp. 159–61.

7. Foudraine, J. (1974), op. cit., p. 164.

8. Foudraine, J. (1974), op. cit., p. 195.

9. Foudraine, J. (1974), op. cit., p. 181.

10. Foudraine, J. (1974), op. cit., pp. 298−9.

11. Foudraine, J. (1974), op. cit., pp. 184, 190, 172, 183, 199.

12. Foudraine, J. (1974), op. cit., Introduction.

13. Foudraine, J. (1974), op. cit., p. 170.

14. Evans-Pritchard quoted in D. Ingleby, 'Understanding "Mental illness"' in D. Ingleby (ed.) (1981) *Critical Psychiatry: The Politics of Mental Health*, p. 26. Harmondsworth: Penguin.

15. Scott, R. D. 'Support groups for hospital staff within the context of dynamic psychiatry', unpublished paper.

16. Foudraine, J. (1974), op. cit., p. 230.

17. Foudraine, J. (1974), op. cit., Introduction.

18. 'Working draft to abolish psychiatry', *Madness Network News* 8 (3) Summer 1986.

19. Georgiades, N. G. and Phillimore, L. (1975) 'The myth of the hero-innovator and alternative strategies for organisational change', in C. C. Kiernan and F. P. Woodford (eds), *Behaviour Modification with the Severely Retarded*. London: Associated Scientific Publishers.

20. Scott, R. D., op. cit.

21. Department of Health and Social Security (1972) Report of the Professional Investigation into Medical and Nursing Practices on Certain Wards at Napsbury Hospital near St Albans. London: HMSO.

22. *Evening Echo*, 26 May 1972.

23. *Evening Echo*, 27 May 1972.

24. *Evening News*, 22 February 1973.

25. *Daily Mail*, 22 February 1973.

26. *Daily Mail*, 22 February 1973.

27. Report of the Professional Investigation into Medical and Nursing Practices (1972), op. cit.

28. *Daily Express*, 22 February 1973.

29. *Evening Echo*, 21 February 1973.

CHAPTER 11

1. Kraepelin quoted in D. Hill (1985) *The Politics of Schizophrenia*. Lanham: University Press of America.

2. Rosenhan, D. L. (1973) 'On being sane in insane places', *Science* 179: 250−8.

3. Ullmann, L. P. and Krasner, L. (eds) (1975) *A Psychological Approach to Abnormal Behaviour*, 2nd Edition, pp. 203−9. Englewood Cliffs, NJ: Prentice-Hall.

4. Orbach, S. (1986) *Hunger Strike*. London: Faber & Faber.

5. Garson quoted in R. Warner (1985) *Recovery from Schizophrenia: Psychiatry and Political Economy*, p. 49. London: Routledge & Kegan Paul.

6. Parsons quoted in G. Baruch and A. Treacher (1978) *Psychiatry Observed*, p. 244. London: Routledge & Kegan Paul.

7. *Guardian*, 3 October 1986.

8. Warner, R. (1985), op. cit., p. 30.

9. *Independent*, Tuesday 4 November 1986.

10. Ratna, L. (1978) 'Crisis intervention in psychogeriatrics: a two-year follow-up study', in L. Ratna (ed.) *The Practice of Psychiatric Crisis Intervention*. Published by The League of Friends, Napsbury Hospital.

11. Department of Health and Social Security (1980) *Inequalities in Health*.

12. Health Education Council (1987) *The Health Divide*.

13. Miles, A. (1981) *The Mentally Ill in Contemporary Society*. Oxford: Martin Robertson, p. 164.

14. Warner, R. (1985), op. cit., p. 37.

15. Strauss and Carpenter quoted in Warner, op. cit., p. 37.

16. Brown, G., Ni Bhrolchain, M., and Harris, T. (1975) 'Social class and psychiatric disturbance among women in an urban population', *Sociology* 9: 225–54.

17. Rutter, M., Cox, A., Tupling, C., Berger, M., and Yule, W. (1975) 'Attainment and adjustment in 2 geographical areas: I — prevalence of psychiatric disorder', *British Journal of Psychiatry* 126: 493–509.

18. Abramowitz, C. V. and Dokecki, P. R. (1977) 'The politics of clinical judgement: early empirical returns', *Psychological Bulletin* 84: 460–76.

Sutton, R. G. and Kessler, M. (1986) 'National study of the effects of clients' socioeconomic status on clinical psychologists' professional judgements', *Journal of Consulting and Clincial Psychology* 54 (2): 275–6.

Hollingshead, A. B. and Redlich, F. C. (1958) *Social Class and Mental Illness*. New York: Wiley.

Myers, J. K. and Bean, L. L. (1968) *A Decade Later: A Follow-Up of Social Class and Mental Illness*. New York: Wiley.

19. Littlewood, R. and Lipsedge, M. (1982) *Aliens and Alienists: Ethnic Minorities and Psychiatry*. Harmondsworth: Penguin.

20. Littlewood and Lipsedge, op. cit., p. 129.

21. Littlewood and Lipsedge, op. cit., p. 65.

22. Ingleby, D. (1981) in D. Ingleby (ed.) *Critical Psychiatry: The Politics of Mental Health*. Harmondsworth: Penguin.

23. Warner, R. (1985), op. cit.

24. Wing, quoted on jacket of Warner, R. (1985), op. cit.

25. Warner, R. (1985), op. cit., p. 72.

26. Warner, R. (1985), op. cit., pp. 132–4.

27. Warner, R. (1985), op. cit., pp. 126, 137, 139.

28. Warner, R. (1985), op. cit., p. 156.

29. Warner, R. (1985), op. cit., p. 189.

30. Warner, R. (1985), op. cit., p. 266.

31. Warner, R. (1985), op. cit., p. 307.

32. Kovel in Ingleby, op. cit., p. 73.

33. Chesler, P. (1971) 'Patient and patriarch', in V. Gornick and B. K. Moran (eds) *Women in Sexist Society: Studies in Power and Powerlessness*. New York: Basic Books.

34. Penfold, P. S. and Walker, G. A. (1983) *Women and the*

Psychiatric Paradox, pp. 128–9. 138. 139; Montreal, London: Eden Press.

35. Warner, R. (1985), op. cit., p. 139.

36. Kovel in Ingleby, op. cit.

37. Jacoby, R. (1975) *Social Amnesia: A Critique of Conformist Psychology from Adler to Laing*. Brighton: Harvester Press.

38. Bloch, S. and Reddaway, P. (1977) *Psychiatric Terror: How Soviet Psychiatry is Used to Suppress Dissent*, p. 204. New York: Basic Books, p. 204.

39. Schrag, P. (1980) *Mind Control*. London: Marion Boyars, p. 109.

40. Bloch and Reddaway, op. cit., p. 249.

41. Ingleby in *Critical Psychiatry*, op. cit.

42. Ingleby in *Critical Psychiatry*, op. cit., p. 39.

43. Who puts medical students off psychiatry? A meting of the Association of Psychiatrists in Training held at the London Hospital Medical College on 6th February 1979, published by Smith Kline and French Laboratories Ltd., 1979, p. 22.

44. Coulter quoted in *Critical Psychiatry*, op. cit., p. 23.

45. Kovel in *Critical Psychiatry*, op. cit., p. 86.

46. Fee, E. (1983) 'Women's nature and scientific objectivity', in M. Lowe and R. Hubbard (eds) *Women's Nature: Rationalisations of Inequality*. Oxford: Pergamon Press.

47. Kuhn, T. S. (1970) *The Structure of Scientific Revolutions*, (2nd Edition). Chicago: University of Chicago Press.

48. Hill, op. cit., p. 152.

CHAPTER 12

1. Brandon, D. (1981) *Voices of Experience: Consumer Perspectives of Psychiatric Treatment*, pp. 16–19. MIND.

2. *We're Not Mad . . . We're Angry!* shown in Channel 4's Mind's Eye season on aspects of mental health and mental illness, Autumn 1986.

3. *Mind's Eye*, pp. 14–16, published by Channel 4 Television, September 1986.

4. Lorion, R. P. (1978) 'Research on psychotherapy and behavior change with the disadvantaged; past, present and future direction', in S. L. Garfield and A. E. Bergin (eds) *Handbook of Psychotherapy and Behaviour Change: An Empirical Analysis*. Chichester: John Wiley & Sons.

5. *Off the Breadline: A Better Life*. MIND Publications.

6. *Off the Breadline: A Better Life*. MIND Publications.

7. Warner, R. (1985) *Recovery from Schizophrenia: Psychiatry and Political Economy*. London: Routledge & Kegan Paul.

8. Braithwaite, J. (1984) *Corporate Crime in the Pharmaceutical Industry*. London: Routledge & Kegan Paul.

9. David Smail in *Changes*, vol. 4, no. 5, October 1987.

Index